Two Faced

THOMAS SEKELIUS

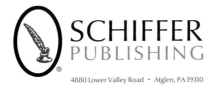

SCHIFFER PUBLISHING

4880 Lower Valley Road · Atglen, PA 19310

Other Schiffer Books on Related Subjects:
Classic Beauty: The History of Makeup, Gabriela Hernandez,
ISBN 978-0-7643-5300-0

Originally published as *two/faced* by Bonnier Fakta, Sweden,
© 2018 Thomas Sekelius
Translated from the Swedish by Simulingua, Inc.
Photos: Emma Svensson, Beata Holmgren,
and Sanna Krantz for Studio Emma
Svensson Graphical form Li Söderberg
Editor: Anna Sodini

Library of Congress Control Number: 2020930849

Cover design by Molly Shields
Type set in Modern No. 20/Telemaque FY

ISBN: 978-0-7643-6050-3
Printed in India

Published by Schiffer Publishing, Ltd.
4880 Lower Valley Road
Atglen, PA 19310
Phone: (610) 593-1777; Fax: (610) 593-2002
E-mail: Info@schifferbooks.com
Web: www.schifferbooks.com

For our complete selection of fine books on this and related subjects, please visit
our website at www.schifferbooks.com. You may also write for a free catalog.

Schiffer Publishing's titles are available at special discounts for bulk purchases
for sales promotions or premiums. Special editions, including personalized
covers, corporate imprints, and excerpts, can be created in large quantities for
special needs. For more information, contact the publisher.

We are always looking for people to write books on new and related subjects. If
you have an idea for a book, please contact us at proposals@schifferbooks.com.

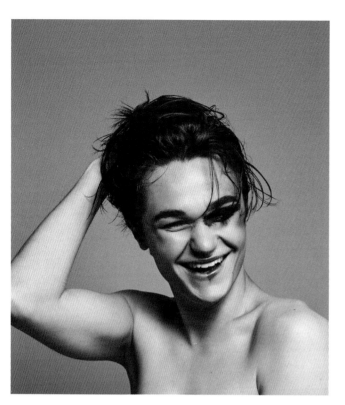
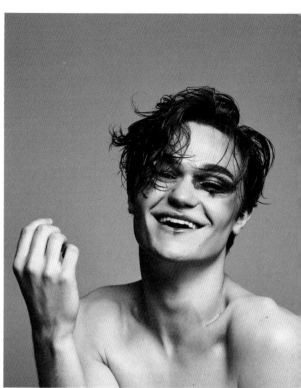
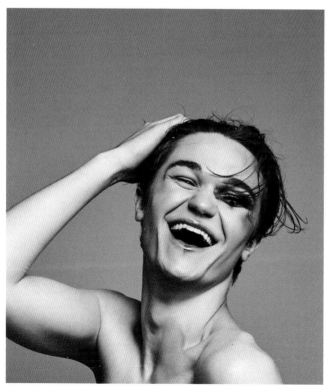
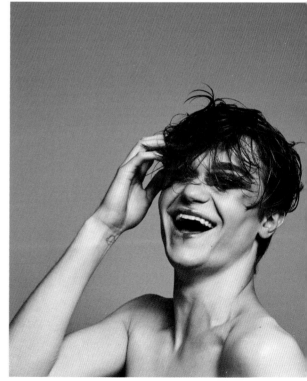

Two faced

All my life I have lived in a society where two rules apply: less is more and makeup isn't for guys. I hope for a place where the "more is more" principle can also apply, and where makeup can be used by everyone.

My path into the wonderful world of makeup went through YouTube and a school musical we did at my *gymnasium*, which is roughly the equivalent of high school in the US. I'd watched a lot of beauty clips online but had never really done a full face of makeup. But now I'd gotten a part in a musical, and before the premiere we had to learn about face shaping theatre makeup (all-natural shadows on your face disappear when you stand there with the spotlights trained on you). I had a jump on how to proceed, thanks to my previous YouTube consumption, but actually had very little practical experience. Mastering makeup is not a quick process and everyone has to make mistakes, but we all have to have a starting point. The makeup studio at school was mine.

I started by doing make up on myself, saw that I hit my stride immediately, and was then completely convinced that that was something I wanted to learn more about. After that first makeup attempt with the school musical, I went straight home and ordered a starter kit with makeup and brushes. It also became the starting point for the blog I wrote for two months, which in turn led me to start posting my own makeup videos on YouTube.

On June 1, 2015, I uploaded my first video, which was called "Introduction"—about me, my channel, and guys who use makeup. It begins with me, unmade up/without any makeup, lipsyncing to Beyoncé and Chimanda Ngozi Adichie's song "Flawless" and follows with me disappearing from the camera and then reappearing with a fully madeup face. I continued with my YouTube clips, bolstered by the encouragement I received from my followers, who quickly grew in number. Meanwhile, my time at gymnasium immediately got a lot more stressful . . .

And now I have written this book in the hope that you too will experience what I feel when I settle down in front of the mirror and lay out palettes, brushes, and pencils. I refer to it simply as my "makeup meditation." I want to emphasize that I am not a trained makeup expert, but what I'm demonstrating here I have learned through practice, practice, practice. And if I can, you can! Because it's just like the saying goes: practice makes perfect. You have to make a lot of mistakes before it gets good.

In this book, "natural" isn't going to be synonymous with "better," and lots of makeup doesn't have to mean "cakey." My point of departure is to write about makeup in a gender-inclusive way, because I know from experience what it's like to be interested in an industry that shuts you out. The idea that makeup should be only for girls is actually quite laughable.

Makeup, just like fashion, is an art form in constant motion, and trends in the use of makeup according to gender affiliation have shifted through history. For example, in ancient Egypt, wearing makeup was a matter of course for both women and men, but the view of makeup in ancient Greece became coded as somewhat feminine. But hopping over to England during the sixteenth century, and makeup was something for everyone regardless of gender. The pendulum swings, and—who knows—maybe something like that is happening right now. Makeup is one size fits all—it's society that has to recognize it.

In this book, I will explain my makeup style and give my best tips, which doesn't have to be the only way to go. The world of makeup is huge, really huge. New brands and products pop up every day, and it is difficult to know which of the 17,245 primers you should choose. It is also easy to get stuck in a style of makeup, and it's obviously hard to try something new, such as false eyelashes, winged eyeliner, or large Instagram eyebrows.

I'd like to challenge you to test one of the following two options in the next week:

1. Before you take off your makeup at night, try a makeup style you've always wanted to try.

2. Before you leave home for the day, try a makeup style you've always wanted to try.

For example, eyeliner is something that a lot of people struggle with. To practice, apply a line as the last thing in the evening before you remove your makeup. If you try and get it wrong, it doesn't matter because you're going to wash it off anyway. If the eyeliner is perfect, it seems like a pity to take it right off, but then maybe it's time to try option two the next day. (Or you can admit defeat, leave the mirror, and hope nobody notices the undercover panda subbing for you at work.) Option 2 is slightly more stressful in the morning, but when you nail it—what a feeling!

For me, makeup isn't something I hide behind, and I urge anyone who feels like they have to wear it every day to try to think the same way. See makeup as something fun, something creative, an art form, or a hobby instead of something that has to adorn your face for your beauty to emerge. The title of the book you hold in your hand reflects to some extent the fact that I try to separate makeup-Thomas and Thomas-Thomas. I see the beauty of Thomas without makeup, and I see the beauty of Thomas with makeup without comparing them. Yes, a face that has just been washed, peeled, face masked, and moisturized, that reminds me of the butt I had when I was two years old, is hard to beat! But a face made up with full coverage foundation, a smokey eye, rosy cheeks, glossy lips, and long lashes makes my heart do somersaults.

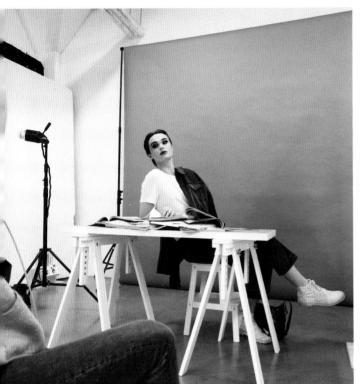
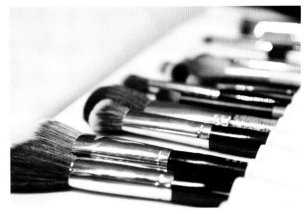
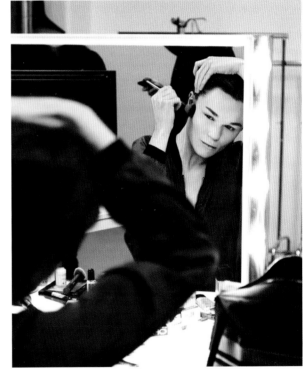
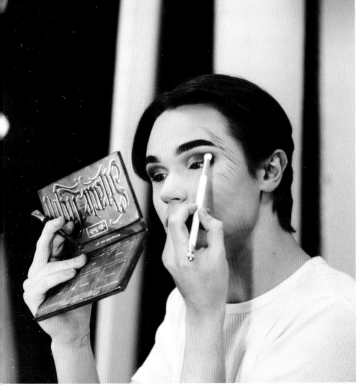
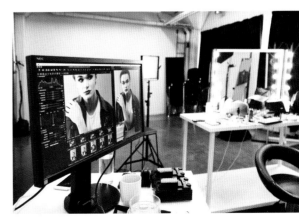

"A face made up with full coverage foundation, a smokey eye, rosy cheeks, glossy lips, and long lashes, makes my heart do somersaults."

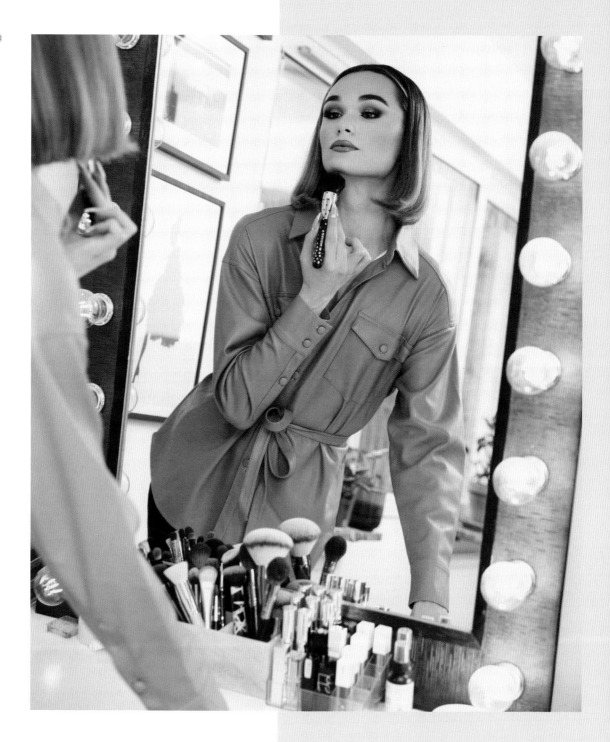

In my makeup bag

As you can probably guess, I have a lot of makeup at home. A shelf in the bathroom cabinet or a toiletry bag wouldn't go too far. Instead I keep most of my makeup in a tall chest of drawers, my makeup pedestal/pillar as I usually call it. Here's a description of the products I use given in the order that I usually use them. At the end, you'll also see how I think when I'm packing for a trip and can't take everything with me.

Brushes and hygiene

A makeup bag can reveal a lot about a person. Are you someone who washes your brushes after every use and never has any expired products and used cotton swabs or pads in your makeup bag? Or are you someone who actually knows that old products and bacteria-filled sponges cause impurities on your face and are always complaining about it while being too lazy to do anything about it? I would put myself somewhere in the middle. I know I should wash my makeup brushes at least once a week, but who manages, remembers, or can justify it, when it takes so long; and they look the same after one use anyway.

To give an example, let's pretend I'm a person who has an angel and a devil on each shoulder. The angel says I should think about the blackhead I squeezed yesterday and how clean brushes might prevent that. The devil counters with the claim that it will take time, I'll probably get my shirt wet, and end halfway through with me regretting it, as my inner laziness gets the upper hand.

It's important to wash the makeup brushes, so that they don't accumulate too much bacteria, but also because they'll last longer, and give a more beautiful application to whatever you put on your face.

Now let's promise each other to try to wash our makeup brushes once a week. It's kinder on both our skin and our wallet!

Primer, foundation, concealer, and powder

I have never been someone who is tied to a particular primer; I just want a base where my pores look as small as possible and my skin gets smooth and ready for foundation. For some reason, some primers don't work well with some foundations. It could be due to any number of things: ingredients that separate when they come into contact with one another, or a skin type that stands in the way of a fine marriage between primer and foundation—you just won't have a good result.

Which type of primer, foundation, and concealer suits you is always very personal and it's best to test several different kinds over a longer period of time. Don't be afraid to replace the products in your makeup bag; what you think suits you might not be what actually does. So test all the products you find.

And to complicate things a little, different combinations of primer, foundation, concealer, and powder work differently for different looks. Sometimes I want to be lightly kissed by coverage and sometimes I want a full on make out session with the thickest, most heavy-duty foundaton I can find.

the eyes—last longer and prevent the product from settling in fine lines, as it sometimes can do under the eyes. Baking also brightens up the places where you apply it. To set and bake your undereyes, take some loose setting powder and press it directly onto the sticky base. Let it sit for up to fifteen minutes, preferably until you have finished your eye makeup. This allows the base to absorb more powder than if you were using a brush, it stays matte longer, and it sits better on the skin. Personally, I use baking to some extent every time I do my makeup. I mattify under my eyes and in the middle of my forehead by pressing firmly with a

Sometimes I want to be lightly kissed by coverage and sometimes I want a full on make out session with the thickest, most heavy-duty foundation I can find.

I have never understood those of you who use foundation and concealer without fixing it with a powder—what do you do during the day? Do you put a dome over your head so you don't leave half of your face on the first person you hug, or to prevent dust from sticking to your sticky, unfixed face?

Jokes aside, I understand you, but I prefer to fix my base. Some people don't put more effort on powder than just slightly fixing their concealer or mattifying the contour area for the shading to easier blend out. The reason is that it gives a more skin-like finish, lets the skin breathe, and keeps you more moisturized. When it comes to mature skin, my advice is to be sparing with the amount of powder you use. It may be good in some circumstances, but can also defeat the purpose and highlight your fine lines.

Baking is also not recommended for mature skin. Baking, or cooking as it is sometimes called, originates from the drag world and became popular not least thanks to internet personalities such as Kim Kardashian, and is used to fix and brighten up your concealer. The purpose of the technique is to make your base more matte—especially the area under

makeup sponge and dust it off right away with a powder brush. In other words, I don't let the powder sit for a long period of time and I don't do it all over my face. This provides a secure fixing without overusing powder, which can sometimes feel tight and dry on your face because of the talc in the powder.

Contour, bronzer, and blush

I switch between a couple of different contour palettes. When talking about eye shadows, you often want high pigmentation, but that's not the goal with contour shadows because that would only make blending more difficult. I focus on the color of the shadow more than the pigmentation when contouring because I am still very careful to build these shadows instead of smearing on a dark spot, thinking that it'll blend into a natural shade. Less pigment means that the shadow needs to be built up; more concentrated pigmentation means the brush will hold more product, which in turn will also be more obvious on your face and, in the worst case, leave you with a patchy, unnatural shadow.

Then comes bronzer and blush, which in my opinion, are a must when contouring; otherwise I

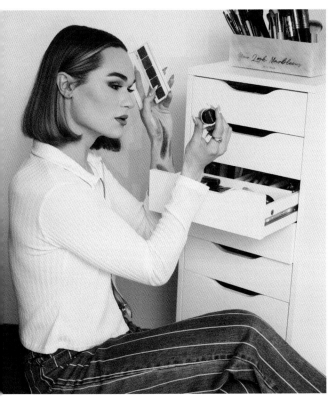
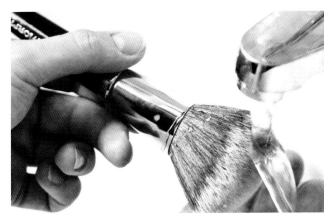
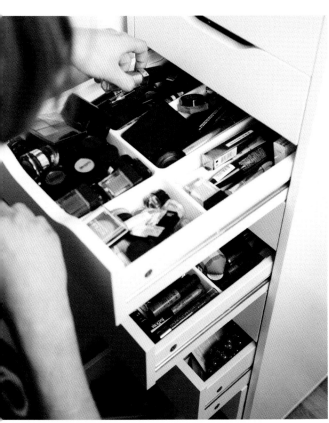
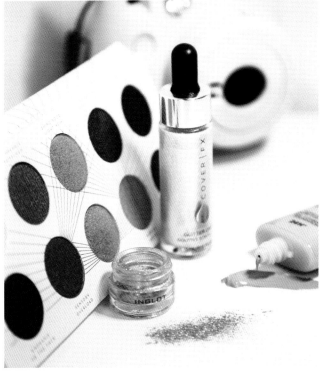
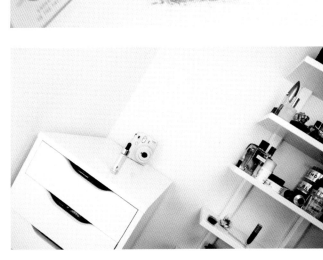

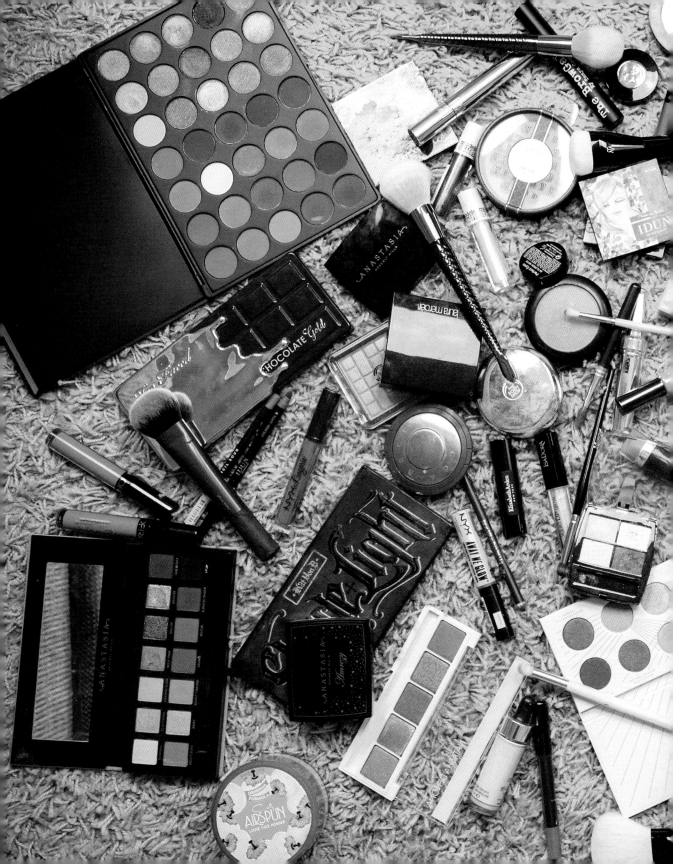

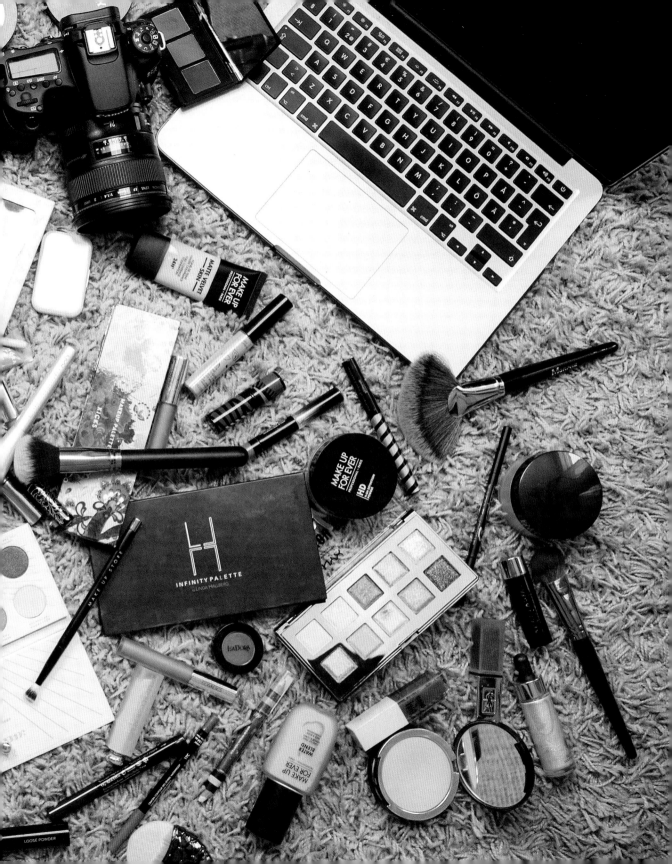

feel dull. If I want to minimize my number of products, there are kits on the market that include bronzer, blush, highlighter, and a cool contour shadow.

Eyebrow pencil and eyebrow pomade

Eyebrow pencil works best for me on my eyebrows, because it is quick and looks the most natural. I should add that when I call makeup "natural," I mean one of two things. Either I mean "natural" in the sense that the illusion that I create looks natural—for example, if I want a full coverage foundation but still want to get the finish to look like skin, not a powdery

between. Mostly I end up somewhere in the middle, starting from a natural palette but realizing halfway through that I'm not satisfied yet, and I dunk my face in holographic glitter.

Usually I have matte eye shadows for the look I'm doing in the same palette, but if I want to have a shimmering lid, eyeliner, or a smokey eye, I'll need some complementary products.

False eyelashes and mascara

A common misconception about false lashes is that they're not reusable. Most lashes can be used from five

A common misconception about false eyelashes is that they're not reusable. Most lashes can be used from five to fifty times, depending on how well you store them, how much glue you apply per use, and if you wash the lashes when they become too covered in mascara.

layer on the skin—or if I create a new shape for my brows but want what I drew outside my natural brow shape to look like my own brows.

When I don't use brow pen, I'll happily use brow pomade instead. For those of you who also like it, I have a trick to make the pomade a little creamier. Some brands have products called mixing liquid. What is does is act as a mixing base for various products. I have one from Inglot which is a little oily in texture which dissolves the pomade, mixes into it, and makes it creamier, waterproof, and allows you to revive an old, dried-out pomade. If you have no mixing liquid, coconut oil works as an alternative.

Eye shadow

I have eye shadows for all types of makeup looks: for colorful, provocative, and crazy looks, for natural, slightly defined, and sexy looks; and everything in

to fifty times, depending on how well you store them, how much glue you apply per use, and if you wash the lashes when they become too covered in mascara.

To wash your false eyelashes, you need two cotton pads and a clean mascara or spoolie brush. To dissolve glue and mascara, place the lashes between the pads and then saturate them in makeup remover. Then you just brush out the mascara that wasn't dissolved with a clean mascara brush, and your lashes are like new.

Lipstick and lip gloss

You get pretty far with a nude (a shade close to your own skin tone) lipstick and a lip gloss, but it's obviously fun to experiment with lip products throughout the color range. Keep in mind that lipsticks can also function as blush or even as eye shadow if you put a little on your fingertip and dab it on.

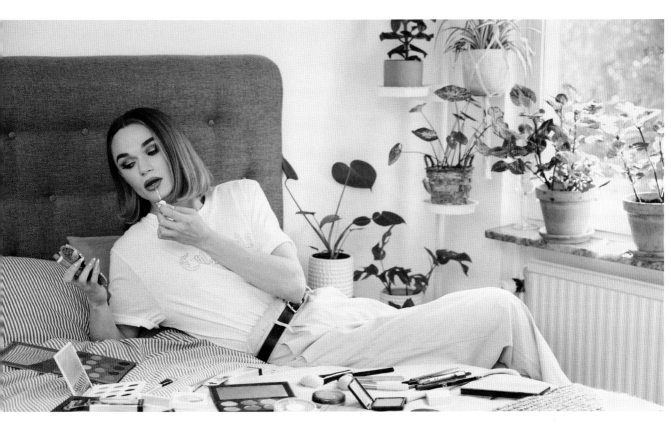

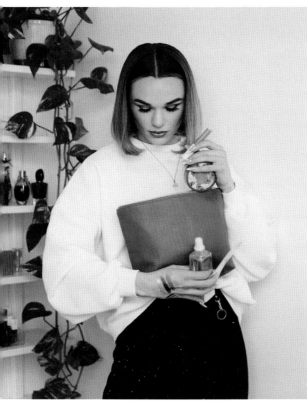

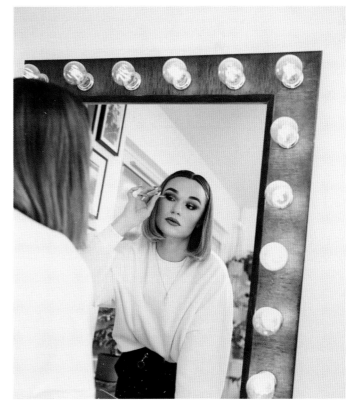

Setting spray or water

When I have created a full-coverage base that I fixed with a lot of powder, I want a setting spray that melts together my powder products with my skin and makes the makeup last longer. When I have lighter bases and don't need to think about the amount of makeup on my face, I spray on some water that gets the powder products to fuse with the liquid on my skin and gives a natural, skin-like appearance.

Pack for the trip

When bringing my makeup on a trip or doing makeup away from home, I always consider the order in which I put the products on my face. I have a tendency to

a base. As for the rest of the face, there are a lot of different ways to put your products to multiple uses. You could pack an eyeshadow palatte that contains a shadow for your brows, you could use your cream blush as lipstick or the other way around, you could use your brow pencil as a soft eyeliner, you could use your contour, bronzer, and highlighter as eyeshadows... Well, you get the picture—just because a product has a specific area that it's made for doesn't mean you have to stick to it. On pages 42–43 I show a step-by-step tutorial on how to do it.

I pack a palette that includes a warm, a cold, and a shimmering brown shadow in order to both create contour and and warm up my face. I even use these

Lipstick can also function as blush or even as eye shadow if you put a little on your fingertip and dab it on..

forget products at home but have realized that if I pack using this method, I usually get everything I need. This trick probably isn't necessary for those with ony a few products in your makeup routine, but for those of us who take two suitcases over when we do makeup at a friend's house, it can be helpful.

At times when I have to bring as little makeup as possible along, but still have the opportunity to do a full face of makeup, I try to pack products that I can use in multiple ways. To minimize the amount of products I also skip as many steps as I possibly can. I do not pack a foundation, only a primer and a concealer. I focus the coverage of the concealer under my eyes, in the middle of my forehead, along my nose and chin area, concentrating the coverage in the middle of my face. This gives the look of a fully covered face, without using too many products. Be sure not to use a super light concealer since you don't have a foundation to balance it out. After this, I like to go in with a cream contour to sculpt my face and to get some more coverage on the perimeter of my face and on the cheeks. This is what works best for me as

colors as eye shadow so I don't have to pack another palette. Because I like to do my brows with a pencil, I put that in my bag, too, but if you prefer powder for your brows, you could even use your contour palette here. If not, I recommend prioritizing an eye shadow palette that contains a shadow you can also use for your brows.

If I have room, I usually put everything I need for the ten possible makeup looks I've planned; I'd rather have too much to choose from than to get the perfect idea that can't be realized because I left the neon pink at home.

At regular intervals I go through which products I packed and check them against my imaginary list to make sure that I haven't forgotten anything, and each time I see that my powder *is* actually in the bag, I relax because it is one of my best friends. Once the lashes are packed, I turn to the lip products where I really don't think beyond having a nude color and a lip gloss with me that I can have as a plan B. As plan A, I just throw in all the colors I think would fit with the color range I chose, and hope for the best.

Makeup for everyone

Regardless of whether you want to cover all your problems with a layer of full-coverage foundation and continue living your best life or sweep a light bronzer over your cheeks, add a few strokes of mascara, and move on with the day, I encourage you to do it your own way, precisely the way you like. Makeup is, in my opinion, an art form and a means of self-expression and nobody does it better than you. Live your makeup dreams to the fullest; over time, self-confidence will come. Not because of the makeup itself, but with the feeling that you look the way you want to, and are 100 percent yourself. Being yourself, and being able to express yourself as you like, is incredibly close to my heart. Let's have one another's backs, include everyone, not just the privileged, open ourselves to discussion, and steer the world to a better place. If you have a voice, use it. Not just for your own profit, but also for the sake of your fellow human beings.

An incredibly important thing for me when it comes to makeup is that brands are not only marketed with the help of slender white girls, but that you work with people of all ethnicities, with varied skin tones, and of different sexes, and make products that match and perform as well in darker tones as they do in lighter ones. There's no order to the brands listed here—they all have good color offerings and product quality is consistent and as promised throughout their range.

Brands that make forty shades of foundation where only twenty of them are the requisite quality, and the rest are only designed only to look good on the store shelves won't fulfill their purpose when bad reviews start spreading online.

In short, more brands should open their eyes and embrace the fact that customers exist in more than six shades, four of which are similar and two are poorly colored shades of orange.

Inclusive brands that are easy to find
- *Fenty Beauty*
- *NYX Professional Makeup*
- *Make Up Forever*
- *Lancôme*
- *Cover FX*
- *Hourglass*
- *Black Opal*
- *La Girl*
- *Il Makiage*
- *Bobbi Brown*
- *Uoma*
- *Hue Noir*
- *Giorgio Armani*
- *Anastasia Beverly Hills*
- *Danessa Myricks*

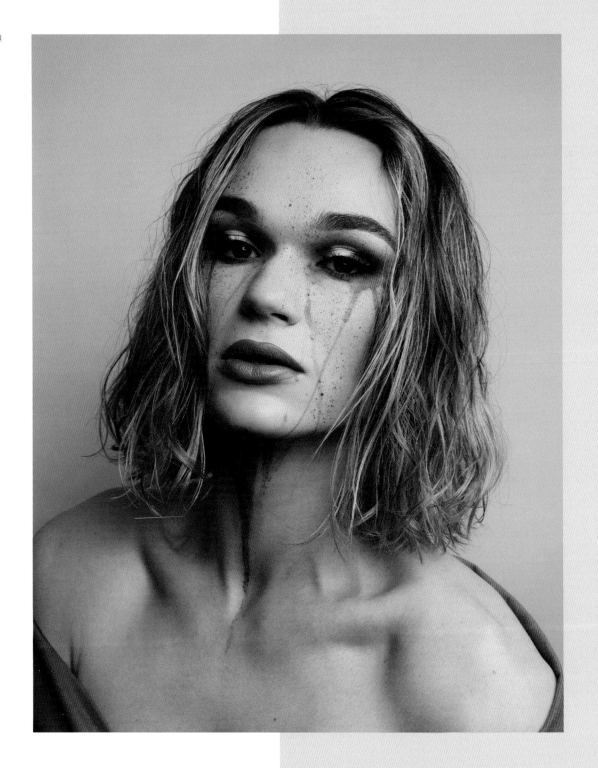

I am transgender

Write. Erase. Write. Erase.

I've been debating with myself for too long on how to start this page in the book, procrastinating to the fullest. Do I write the full story, do I focus on how I feel regarding the matter today, or do I try to summarize the confusing whirlwind of thoughts that is roaming around in my mind at all times? I've come to the conclusion that the latter is the most honest way to go, since I am still at the very start of my life-changing journey and am still figuring things out.

Write. Erase. Breathe. Collect thoughts.

I was a rather norm-fitting child, doing what society wanted me to, but always open to try what intrigued me, whether it was getting a new toy car or trying on my mom's leather boots that she wore once and then buried in the back of the closet for me to occasionally risk the health of my ankles in. If I saw something that interested me, I wanted to try it. And isn't every young mind similar in this behavior? I believe that when we are born, our minds are open to anything that makes us happy or that interests us in any type of way, until shame and division are applied to our upbringing. Children get put into a box on the basis of their gender to stay within their stereotypes and never to act otherwise. When constantly getting fed with this information, and the older we get, the way we live is altered to fit this frame. Picture me, a young child, sitting on the floor of the kindergarten playroom. I see a toy truck and I see a toy hairdresser kit next to each other. I crawl up to them, look at them while processing what toy excites me the most, and finally pick the latter. If I then get a comment that shames me or tries to change my decision, I will think twice when choosing my next toy. This can be applied to a whole lot in our youth and limit us to what might have been if we were actually encouraged to act on our desires. Instead of doing what we love, we try to fit into the blueprint of what society has molded into being the ideal, whether that be what interests we pursue, what clothes we wear, how we behave, or what decisions we make. We become questioning, skeptical, and hesitant and take distance from what we deep-down know we are destined to do, what to wear or how to express ourselves, and instead take an easier way, canceling out any hardships that may occur by taking the path that isn't approved by society. Of course there are exceptions of the greater mass, but they're sadly a rarity until later in life. I for instance wasn't able to find my true self until the age of sixteen, when I started a new school.

Write. Erase. Get emotional. Cry.

When I started high school, or the gymnasium as we call it in Sweden, I began my first journey of finding myself while trying to manage my newly surfaced eating disorder and self-harm. This was a time of being broken down and experiencing growth at the same time. I accepted the fact that I was gay and started working on overcoming my internalized homophobia, I made new friends, I started to blossom as a person, and I did what I truly wanted to do. My mind, however, was running hot with body dysmorphia, self-hatred, anxiety, and suicidal thoughts. I just hated myself, but I never really knew why; I just did, especially my body.

Write. Erase. Reminisce. Collect thoughts.

Time went by, I got older, I got into social media and makeup, and I could finally breathe and feel relief from my troubled mind as I felt happier, more energized, and full of purpose, something that I had been lacking for so long. However, I could not for the life of me escape the distorted image of myself. Sure, it got a lot easier, but I don't know if it was

because I truly was in a better mindset, because I focused all my energy on my job, or because feeling this way had been the standard for me for so long that I got used to it.

After a few years of me wearing makeup and having a feminine approach to self-expression, I started to notice a new feeling in the mixture of self-hatred, a feeling that finally gave me some answers or at least a red thread to follow in trying to understand my mind. I came to the realization that I was gender fluid, meaning that some days I felt female, and some days I was accepting of the body that I was in. This is a very confusing sensation, and I didn't acknowledge it at first. I thought it was just my aesthetic expression that varied, as it does for a lot of people. I later came to realize that it had to do with my identity as a person, not what I wear and how I look.

During this perplexing period of time, I fell in love. I fell in love with a girl, and what I thought I knew about myself got turned upside down again. Not because of the relationship, which is to this day one of the most beautiful things I've ever experienced, and I am so happy I got to experience that with her, but because I lost myself in overthinking my sexuality and gender identity. Even though I time after time got reassured that I was seen as only me, without any gendered labels, getting full support and respect for my confusion and gender fluidity, I got in my head over being the "boyfriend," the "man." Our relationship was always very gender neutral and I felt so secure, but from an outside perspective I was seen as a boyfriend and was often put in very masculine roles by people who didn't know my situation.

This led me to have to face what was always in the back of my head but that constantly got suppressed subconsciously—my being transgender.

The feeling of my gender identity being fluid changed over time. My acceptance of my masculine body faded and my feminine identity took over completely. The constant urge to change my body and of hating my genitalia, never relating to boys, and being happy when someone said I looked feminine all boiled down to me being transgender. It took me some time to understand what I was constantly trying to change, and once I understood everything that comes with a transition, it hit me like a bus. I started drinking too much to cope with feeling insane by not being ready to start the journey that I knew I had to make to live my life as the real me. My true authentic self. I cried almost every night. Everything that I had been feeling regarding my body suddenly made sense, and it wasn't a dark hole of unexplainable anxiety anymore. It was all very overwhelming, but I also felt relieved. Relieved that I had gotten to a point where I understood why I felt jealous of women, why I tried to achieve female body standards, why I hated the size of my feet, and why I felt more comfortable the more feminine I looked, even though that included tight corsets and an uncomfortable tucking of my genitalia. Everything was worth it, as long as I felt like the true me, which is female.

I first came out a little more than a year ago. The first person I told was my ex-girlfriend, whom I mentioned earlier. I then battled with a lot of internalized transphobia, trying to turn over every rock to see if there was an easier way out of the whirlwind that was my mind. There wasn't. I hated the fact that I was in this position, and I felt angry, sad, and scared. After processing these feelings, I started telling more and more people, while still figuring things out and learning new things about myself everyday. I went through every single scenario I could possibly come up with, feeling my heart beating in my throat when I was about to tell, but then came to realize that my friends are all very accepting and adapted to the situation with open arms. After the first three, four friends, it got a lot easier.

However, this brings me to another conflict I had with myself. The constant need to satisfy the people around me, even if it means I have to compromise what I truly want to do.

Knowing that I wanted to transition, I still tried to persuade myself and others around me that I just didn't want to be put in a masculine position, that a pronoun change was very far into the future, and that I was still figuring things out, which I was, but not regarding that matter. I did this for others not to feel uncomfortable or having to adjust to a new name or a new pronoun, but it was all in my head, and it caught up with me. The feeling of hating the body you're in because you weren't born into the right one is too strong of a feeling. You feel trapped. You feel like you're wearing skin that isn't yours. I couldn't suppress that for too long.

Feeling the need to adapt to what I think other people want me to do is something I'm still working on overcoming. It's hard when it has become a part of you, and I have come a long way, but there is much more to go.

The last step in telling the people who are closest to me was telling my family. The night before I took the train home, I was up until 3 a.m., drinking and bawling my eyes out. I was so scared and nervous, and, sadly, alcohol was my way of coping with breakdowns like this. I again made up every single scenario I could think of, remembering every horrid story I had heard regarding trans people coming out.

I knew my sister would be accepting—there was no doubt—but I was worried for my mom and dad. They're divorced, so I had to do it twice. I sat down at my mom's kitchen table, having already told my sister moments earlier on the terrace, held my sister's hand, and came out to my mother. She had already made herself comfortable with the thought; somehow she knew, and she was fully supportive. I just sat there and cried.

My dad had a worse reaction, giving away a sigh of disappointment when I told him, then giving me a shoulder hug and saying I will always be his Thomas after I told him about a possible name change. However, after I brought it up, he said he meant it as I will always be his child, and that his love for me is stronger than him needing to oppose me. Then we talked about how he has always felt a very "feminine energy" from me.

I am so thankful for having parents who put me first, even if their opinions haven't always been aligned with mine. When I came out as gay, we had some arguments, but I was always very keen on educating them, because I saw that there was a will in them to understand. This is the same situation. Sure, I think my dad will take a longer time than my mom, but as long as he isn't opposed, I can live with it.

There are so many stories on trans people being disowned when coming out, like many others of the LGBTQIA+ community have experienced. Please, don't be that parent. When you have a child, you have the responsibility to always be there for them, within reason. Having a norm-breaking gender identity is not unreasonable. It might take some time to get used to, but it is not out of reason. No, you do not "lose a son or a daughter"—you get one, and a much-happier child. That should be what matters. Skip the "Have you ever thought about how this feels for me?" and focus on trying to understand what it is that bothers your child. Don't see it as something to drive you apart; see it as something that makes you get to know them better.

If you are the child of parents who will accept their child only as heterosexual and cis, remember that as LGBTQIA+ people, we sometimes have to choose our family, and I promise you that there is a family out there, waiting to love and accept you for who you are.

You can't change who you are, and you shouldn't have to. Just be yourself, because there truly is no greater feeling.

Life for me is only beginning. The next chapter is here, and it's a big leap. I just built up the courage to seek help and am on the waiting list to see a doctor. I feel like I'm on the right path in my personal life and am trying to let go of compromising myself to suit others better. I work on loving myself everyday, even though it's hard, and I try to focus on the excitement of my transitioning instead of the hardships it can and will bring. I have not yet come out to the public, but when this book is out, I will either already be out or doing it right now.

BASES

A good base is a base that I don't want to wash off after a couple of hours. It should settle nicely, not get cakey or react with my primer, and last a long time.

Finding the right base combination can take a long time and you might think that the one you are currently using is the one that works, until you test a new foundation, are sold on it, and use it for the next two years. It's like you find your darling and you're loyal until a better one pops up. A bit like dating.

A bad base isn't always the result of bad products. If you have oily skin that you cover with something meant for dry skin, you can get super greasy quickly, because hydrating foundations are for skin that needs moisture. If you have dry skin and use something matte, your skin will react differently.

In this chapter I go through two bases and contouring, or shading, as it is also called.

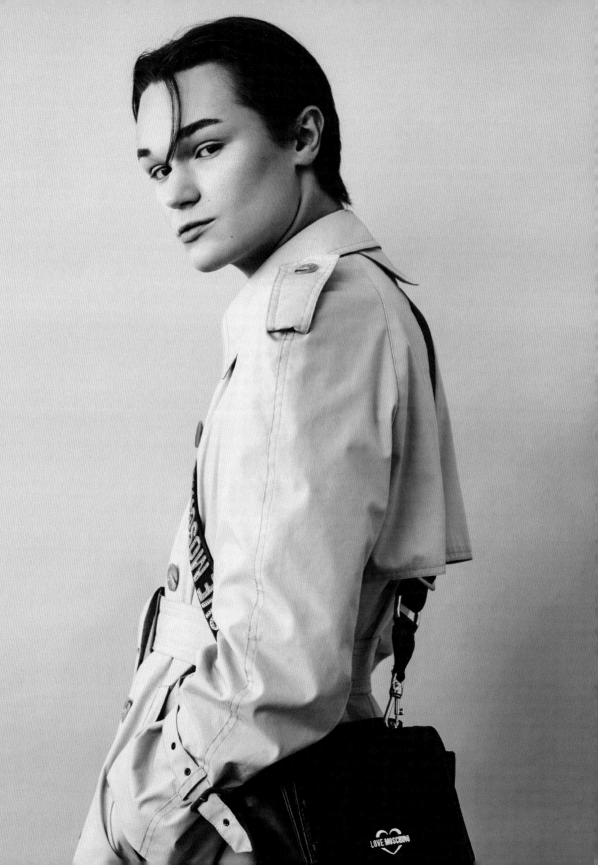

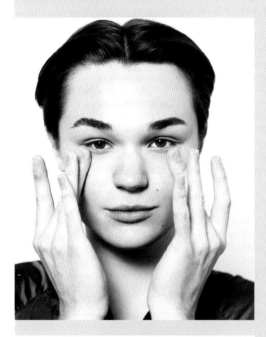

Base 1: Light coverage

For days when you just want to enhance your facial structure, get a confident look with slightly fuller eyebrows, and look a little fresher with some well-placed sweeps of shimmer. I could compare this base with the famous "pregnancy glow" or the way skin can look after a face peeling. There are a few ways to get this look. This one is just a simpler, more controlled, and 100 percent fake way.

STEP 1

Always keep in mind that your skin is your canvas. A primer can never replace moisturized and well-maintained skin. I start with a primer suited to my skin type, so that the makeup will settle better during application and last longer during the day. I have combination skin so I focus a matte primer on the T zone and prime the rest of the face with my moisturizing cream. A good trick is to use a primer that leaves the skin a little moist, because the next step is based on powder.

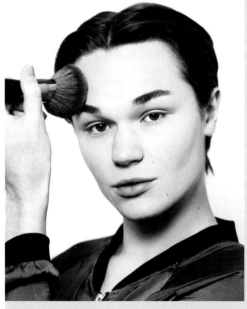

STEP 2

To get very light coverage without having to dilute a liquid foundation and have more product on my face, I use a powder foundation on a large powder brush. The powder evens out my skin tone and provides a base ready to be shaped. For extra coverage under the eyes, I put on some powder foundation with a damp sponge. The sponge concentrates the pigment and doesn't spread it as much as the brush does.

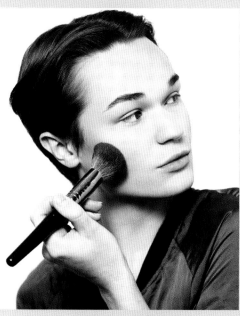

STEP 3
The third step is contouring, which emphasizes, warms up, and reproduces the shape of your natural shadows on your face (read more on page 30). Here I put more focus on blush and bronzer and not so much on sculpted shading.

STEP 4
Finally, I sweep a shimmering powder over the highest points of my face, like the cheekbones, nose, Cupid's bow, chin, and forehead, and then seal all powder products with a couple of pumps of setting spray.

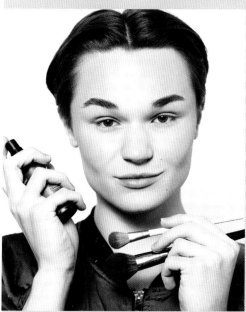

Tips!
A cheaper alternative to setting spray is plain water in a spray bottle.

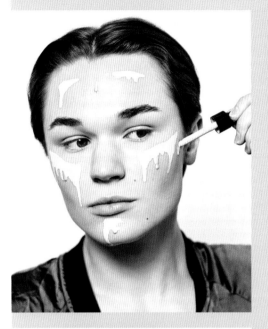

Base 2: Medium coverage

When I want more coverage on my face, I start the look off with a medium coverage foundation that I usually mix with another foundation to get all the benefits from both bases for as controlled a cake face as possible. You can get this look with any level of coverage, and the following is what I prefer.

STEP 1

Here I start with a liquid foundation that I mix with a liquid highlighter to get some extra glow when the natural oils of the skin mix with the powder. Use a sponge for application and don't forget your neck.

STEP 2

Time for concealer. I wear this for two reasons. Partly to brighten up and highlight the high points of the face, and partly for additional coverage. I fix it with a thick layer of transparent loose powder. This process is called "baking."

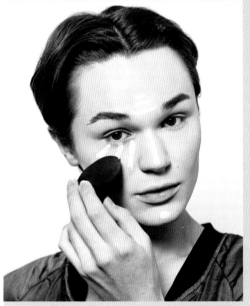

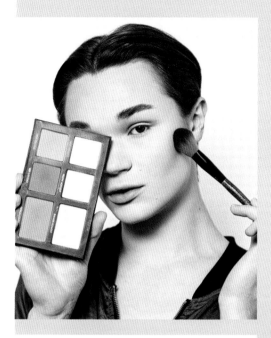

STEP 3

I put a cool contour shadow under my cheek-bone, at the temples, along the sides of my nose and on my jawline. The fuller coverage my base has, the more I shape my face with shadows to regain and emphasize my face shape in a natural way.

STEP 4

Finally, I blend together my slightly cooler contour shadow with a warm, shimmering bronzer and blush, which gives a nice transition from the contouring and gives a warm glow. I apply the highlighter after the bronzer and blush as icing on the cake.

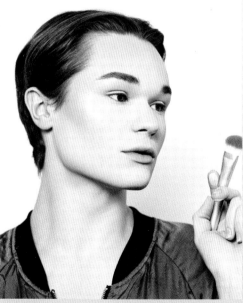

Tips!

Remember to even out your highlighter with the bronzer brush a little to create an invisible transition.

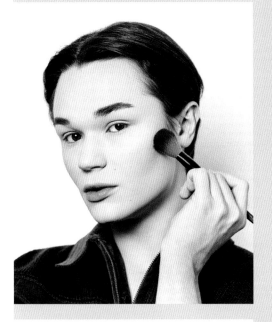

Contouring

Contouring my face is one of my favorite steps in my makeup routine. I see my face re-emerge, take on different looks, ranging from pouty lips to a Tyra Banks smize, while a soft brush massages my face. Which contour shades suit your face, where to place them, and how much to apply, isn't so easy to answer. I've made every mistake you can imagine—too orange, too dark, too gray, not enough blending. But today I can say that I'm sure of my face and could apply a Kim K contour in my sleep. Here's some guidance on how you can go about contouring and I hope that after a little practice you, too, will get to know your face.

STEP 1

The most important thing for me is to build the shadow. I'd rather dip my brush four times than once because the result is smoother and more natural. Here I start with my cheekbones and apply the shadow with small circular movements.

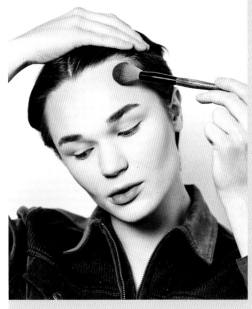

STEP 2

A simple rule to follow is: brightness highlights, shadow conceals. This means that the area you apply your contour color to will look smaller. I have a fairly large forehead, so I put more focus on the temples and hairline.

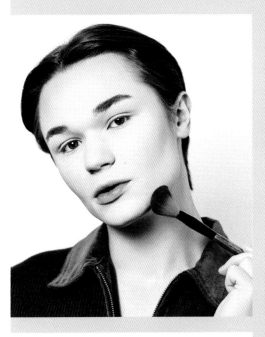

STEP 3

I contour my jaw and nose lightly with what's left on the brush and make sure to apply a little on my neck to make the transition as smooth as possible.

STEP 4

For me it is very important that there is a good balance in my face, that everything is well blended, and that my contouring does not consist of two excessively marked cheekbones.

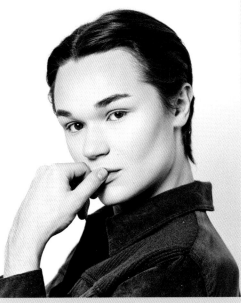

Tips!

Find your contour line. Imagine a line from the corners of your mouth to the middle of your earlobe (the little flap)—this is where you should put your contour. Imagine you draw a big "three" on your face in profile: from the temple, toward the mouth and finish at the jawline—that's your contour template.

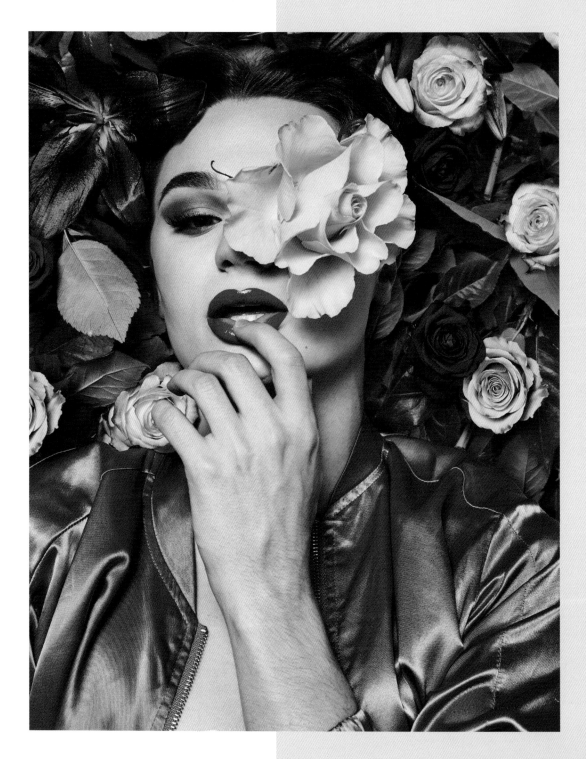

Family and friends

I remember when I was little I had thoughts that felt too big to fit in my head, but luckily I was born with a big head and could start pondering the meaning of life at a young age. "What is the meaning of life?" I asked Mom, who wondered a little about why I was thinking about it. I just couldn't figure out what the meaning of life was and whether or not it was to constantly be seeking joy, love, and striving for the next step in your career.

After a while my mother said soothingly that the meaning of life is whatever *is* meaningful to you. She went on to say that the older I got, the more sure I would be about what was important in my life and my priorities would come from that. Today, at twenty, I can say that family, friends, and the right to be myself all the time are three of my highest priority areas.

My family has supported my choices ever since I was a kid. When my interest in makeup started, I was seventeen years old. I put together ten products online and went with a small lump in my throat to ask Dad for his credit card, because I couldn't use mine online. Instead of asking a lot of questions, we just ordered the stuff. I felt such a relief that my interest did not make him question me. With this little scene I want to illustrate how important it is to have the space to flourish according to your own inner sense and not according to the opinions and norms of other people and to thank my mother, father, and sister, for raising me the way they have and for always having my back and helping me up when I crashed.

In middle school, I tried to fit in with different friend groups and couldn't relax until I got home from school. I tried to dress like everyone else—but I had other ideas and behaved in a way that wasn't really me. It was so strenuous to try to be like others wanted. During the last semester of my ninth year, I developed an eating disorder and I could not pretend anymore. I was completely exhausted. It was hard enough to hide my worrying relationship with food.

Then when I started high school, I could finally relax. I was in a class where everyone put a lot of value on being themselves. I was still afraid to talk about my eating disorder and about my scarred body. After a year, I gathered my courage and went to school in a short-sleeved shirt, showing the scars on my arm. No one said anything until after the first lesson, when some people came up to me and I told them about what had been going on with me, but it wasn't something I wanted to focus on. My interests, makeup, and YouTube were embraced by the class.

The friends from high school are still around, but we don't see each other as often anymore. We all ended up in different places, but sometimes we meet when we are in the same city. My friends are those people who can calm me when I'm anxious; they make me smarter, they question my bad habits; they are always there no matter what I come up with, and they will hopefully always stand by my side, as I stand by theirs.

This makeup includes warm tones that represent the love I feel for my friends and my family. I love you.

EYES

<u>We've all heard that the eyes are the windows to the soul. I would say it's more that the eyes are the part of the face that can be varied most, and that challenge me most creatively.</u>

There are so many eye shadows in infinite color combinations, which in turn are divided into categories by finish. It is usually at this stage that my makeup can go from "natural princess" to a phoenix when I get a glimpse of a red eye shadow that could adorn my entire eye.

Eye shadow is simply the finishing touch to most makeup looks and often takes up a lot of my attention. Here I go through some eye makeup looks with different difficulty levels which will give most of you an opportunity to try and develop your own style!

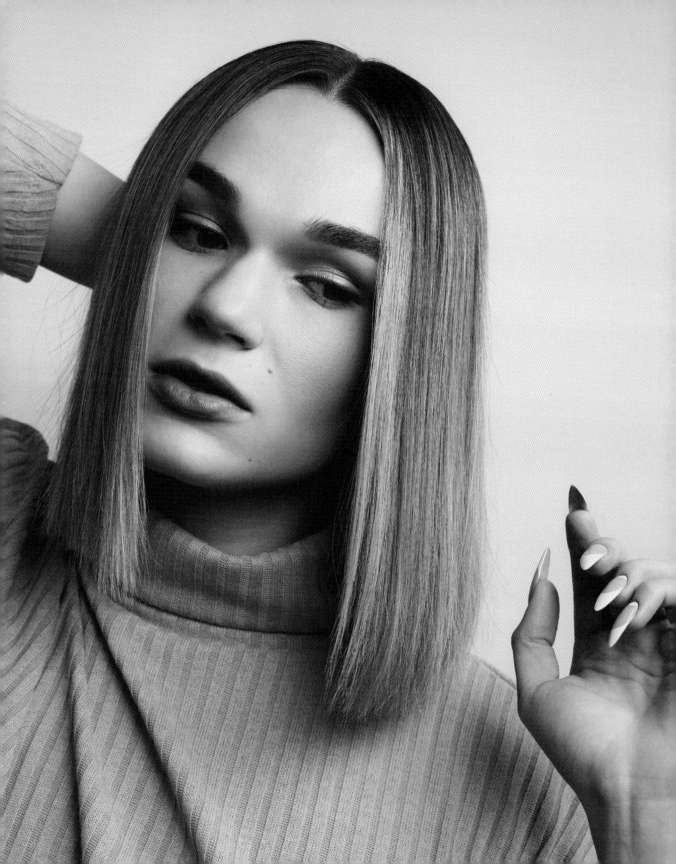

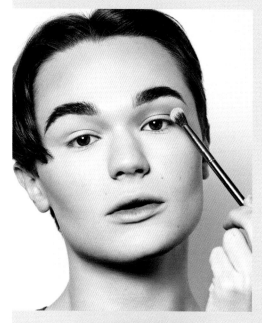

Classic Black Smokey Eye

A timeless eye makeup. The transition color can be replaced by any color, so the combinations to make it more modern are endless.

STEP 1
Building a transition color is important. This is so the black shade won't blend out to an uneven gray tone but instead have a smooth transition. Here I start with an off-white, a light brown, and an orange-brown shade. The goal is that it should be darkest at the crease, where the shadows meet, and then blended out to off-white toward the brow bone.

STEP 2
I continue with a darker-brown shadow and build up even more depth in the crease to ensure a nice transition from black to brown. I work the shadow in small circular motions (the closer to the crease that you put the shadow, the smaller the brush and less movement).

STEP 3
I apply a base of gel eyeliner over the entire eyelid with a flat brush. This ensures that the black eye shadow will stick better and be as dark as possible.

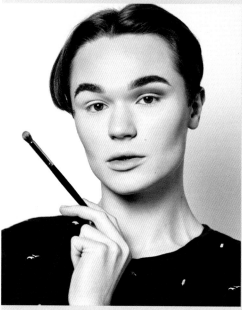

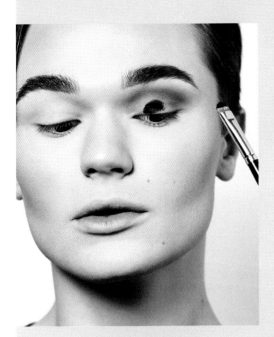

STEP 4

Now I fix the gel line with my black eye shadow. Then I blend together the edges keeping it darkest in the crease. Work with a small brush, to avoid panda eyes.

STEP 5

In the last step, I add my transition color along the lower lash line and then some gel eyeliner. I fix it the same way as I did the eyelid. Don't forget to blend the outer corner together with the rest of the eyeshadow to tie the look together. Just like you need to find out how to contour your own face in the best way for you, everyone's eyes are different. I like to have a lift for a little extra catlike look in my shadow because it suits my eyes best.

Finally, I add a shimmer in the inner corner of the eye to open the eye because black can easily make the eye look smaller.

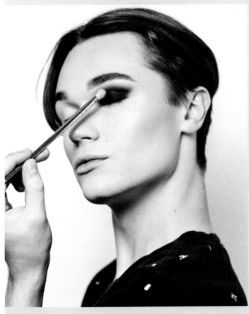

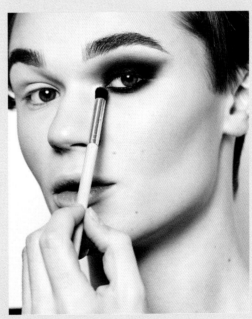

Black shading

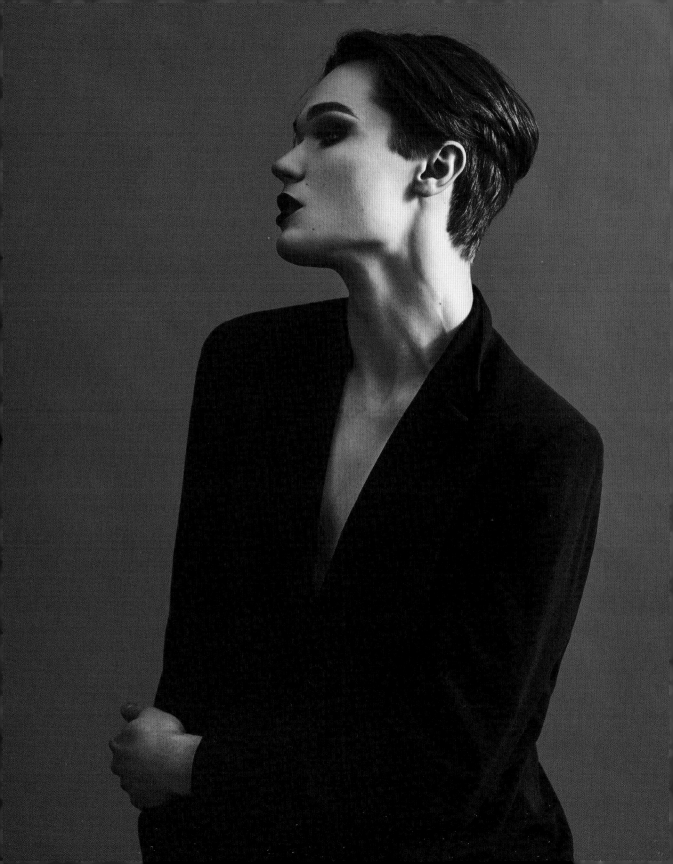

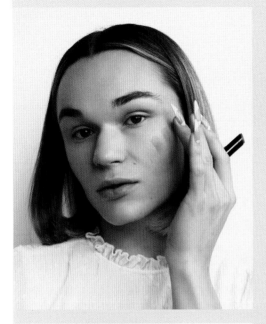

Minimal amount of product

For the times when you can't bring more than a small toiletry bag for your make-up, are in a hurry or simply want your products to have a multi-use purpose, here's some tips and tricks to make things easier for you without having to compromise the finished look.

STEP 1

Skip the foundation and do directly onto concealing. I focus this on my under eye area, forehead, nose and chin. Leave your blush at home and bring with you a creamy lipstick. It works perfectly as a blush! Here I dab a small amount on my cheeks before setting my base and blend it out with either a brush or my fingers.

STEP 2

I contour my face as I normally would and use the same powder with a fluffy blending brush as an eyeshadow to give my crease some depth. You could place this on the lid as well for a brown smokey eye. In addition to highlighting my face, I decided to also place this on my lid for a shimmering look.

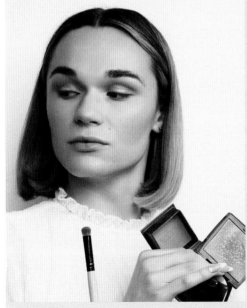

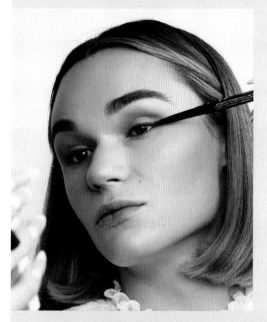

STEP 3

After filling my brows in as described on page 49, I use the same pencil to do a smoked out eyeliner by drawing it along my lash line and blending it out with a small brush. Brown eyeliner is perfect for defining your eyes without making it too intense.

STEP 4

I apply mascara to my lashes and use the same lipstick as I used for my blush to give my lips some color and shine. I didn't want a sharp lip line, so I applied the lipstick in the centre of my lips and blended it out with my ring finger.

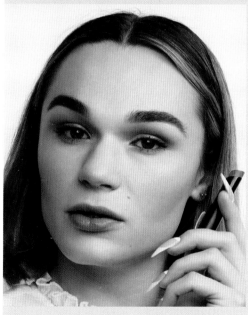

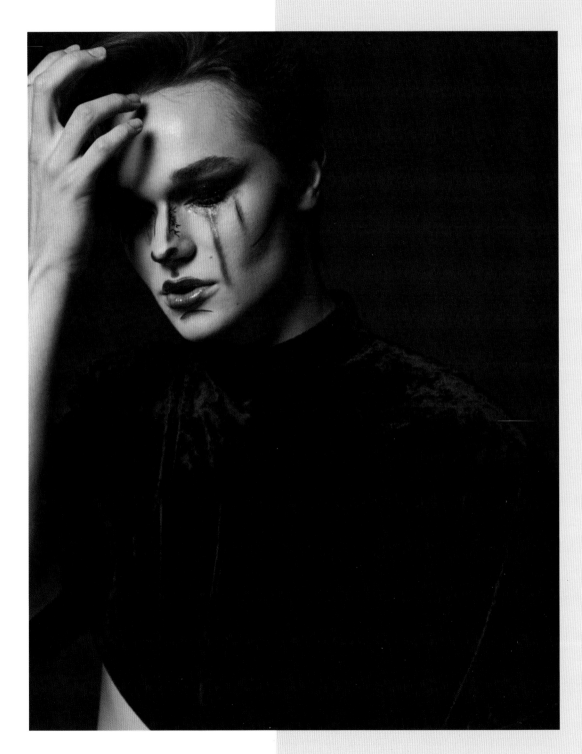

Mental illness

My body issues emerged pretty early. I don't think I'll ever know why. The issues were manageable, though they haunted me and gave me a skewed idea of what I saw in the mirror. I don't remember how, but I stumbled onto an app that could document the calorie content of everything I ate by weighing the food and entering the numbers in the app's system. I became obsessed with this app and realized that a lower calorie intake leads to faster weight loss, and that's what I wanted! The effect was that I first fell ill with bulimia, which then became a mixture of anorexia and bulimia. I starved myself and threw up the food if I failed.

This went on for six months, later accompanied by depression and self-harm in the form of physically injuring myself with sharp objects. For me, self-harm was a bad method of escaping my demons and anxiety, and is an addiction I wouldn't wish on anyone.

When it became bad enough that I could no longer hide my habits from my parents, I told them everything from start to finish, at the dinner table. Dad sat opposite me and mother next to him. I told them that I had a hard time with food and about the self-harming behavior, and asked for help for the first time. I am so glad that their reaction to my horrible news was not anger or assigning blame. That would've just made me feel worse and shut me down even more. Instead, we went to the counselor at school. After some diagnoses and consultations, I started on dialectical behavioral therapy developed for people with emotionally unstable personality disorders.

When I started going to the BUP (Child and Youth Psychiatry Ward), I thought everything was ludicrous/laughable. I didn't understand the point of mindfulness—like imagining a tiger and observing how it moves, or why you should "surf" on your feelings. Now these are the two methods that I remember best and use the most.

Although I feel much better today, I still have some anxiety. The difference is that I have learned to manage it, and that I think it's okay to not always feel good. I think my healing process was accelerated thanks to my YouTube channel. Suffering from mental illness and having symptoms of mental illness is nothing to be ashamed of or something that should be judged. If you suffer from mental illness, keep in mind that you are not weak for asking for help, nor for believing that nothing anyone can say will help you.

For those of you listening to someone speaking out about their difficulties for the first time and putting their trust in you, don't be ridiculing, degrading, or diminishing. Opening up about such a private and vulnerable subject requires a lot of courage and confidence in you as the listener.

If a person gets to talk at their own pace and in their own way, they can explain what they're going through, and then their confidence in the listener is strengthened. If a person is instead met wtih resistance and a dismissive attitude,they'll retreat, lose courage, and it can be hard to muster it up again.

This makeup represents my anxiety in an abstract and fashionable way. Go to hell, anxiety.

EYEBROWS

Here the saying "practice makes perfect" really applies. It is important which techniques you use, but the most important thing is that you think that your brows look good, whether it is a very simple one, a slightly more defined one, or so-called Instagram brows.

My eyebrow journey started a bit before my makeup interest took off. I remember when I was in the makeup department for the first time; I circled nervously around the shelves, went to the eyebrow pencils, and ran into a problem: color. My eyes scanned the pencils, which were clearly marked with brow liner, and eventually stopped on a dark brown that felt like a good match. I went home, tore off the packaging, and tried to fill in my eyebrows for the first time. Guess how it ended?

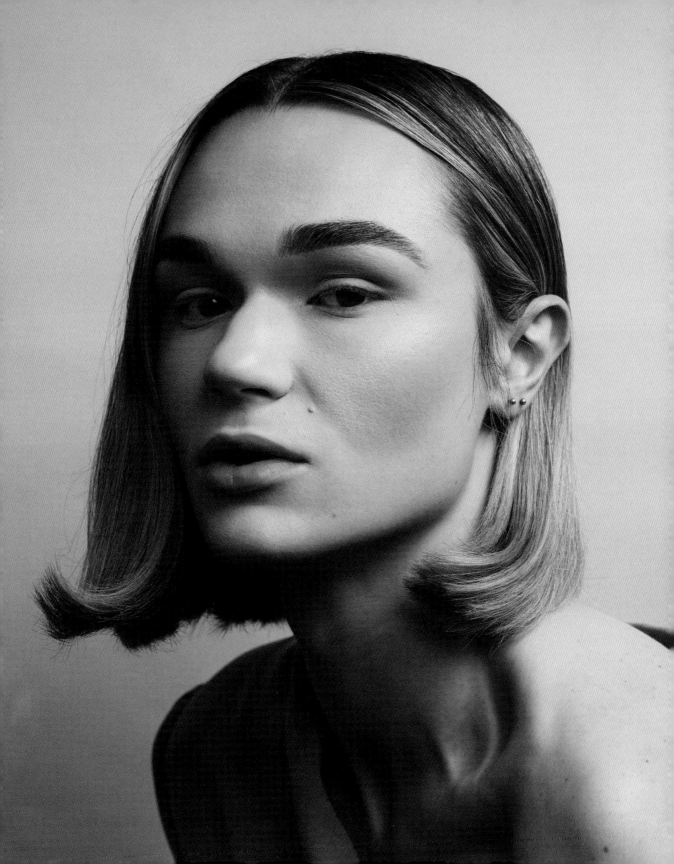

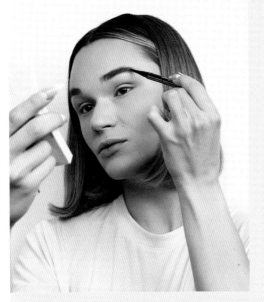

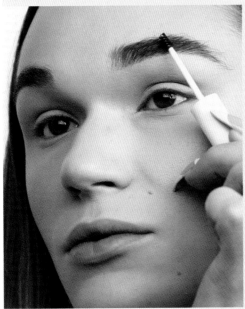

Minimalistic

There are few makeup books that don't have some version of the following sentence: The eyebrows frame the face. This makeup book will not be an exception. The eyebrows really do frame your face.

I knew this, but it became so obvious when I started playing with the shape and color of my eyebrows and realized that my expression and almost the entire face shape could vary, simply because of the eyebrows.

I am a bit of a skincare nerd too, which is sometimes reflected in the way I do my makeup. When I make a light base with a lot of focus on skin, glow, and freshness, I paint these eyebrows. They don't take the focus from my skin but give my face a nice frame.

STEP 1
The first step is to fill in any gaps you might have in your brows. I use a brow pencil that I apply in upward motions, following my natural brow shape.

STEP 2
Once I'm happy with the shape, I make sure to set it with a brow gel. Since the brow is lightly filled in, the way your hairs lie shapes your brow as well, and gives a cleaner look.

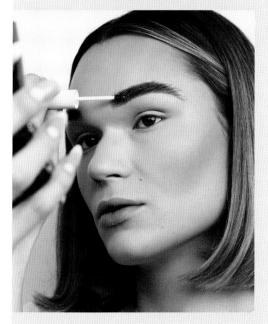

My favorite brows

When you want somewhat bushier eyebrows and a head-to-toe glamorous look without distracting from the rest of the spackled beauty.

STEP 1

I start by brushing my brow hairs down to easier be able to draw hairlike strokes in a downward motion. I draw them a bit outside my natural brow shape for a lifted, more arched look. Then I brush the hairs up and continue filling in the brow with tiny strokes. This gives a more natural look, instead of doing a block of color, as seen in the "Instagram brow".

STEP 2

When the brow is filled in, I extend the tail and make it a bit sharper. Since my brows are far apart, I like to extend the beginning as well by making hairlike strokes in an upward motion, to mimic brow hairs. Top off with brow gel to fixate the brow hairs.

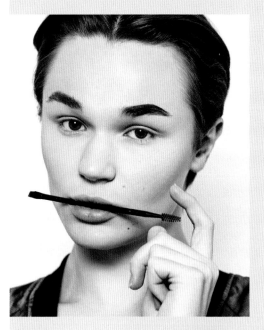

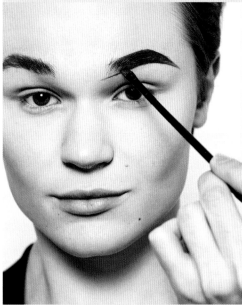

Instagram brows

These brows are the sharpest and most cocky of all. When makeup on Instagram started, a lot of people started to be influenced by the techniques used by drag queens for a long time, such as baking and this more extreme type of eyebrow to lift the whole face and get a tight look.

STEP 1
I start with filling in the outlines of how I want my brow to look, this time with a brow pomade to get as sharp and precise lines as possible.

STEP 2
I fill in the whole brow with the pomade and extend it at the "tail" and in toward the middle. It's better to draw the end of your eyebrows lightly upward rather than downward, because a downward-pointing tail makes your face look droopy.

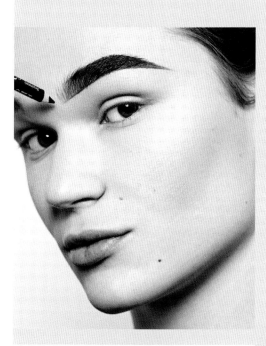

STEP 3

In order to achieve the look I'm after, I use the ombré technique; that is, lightest toward the nose, and getting gradually darker at the end. Then I make small hairlike lines toward the middle to extend the brow and give it a bit bushier and more natural expression.

STEP 4

Finally, I apply a light concealer under the brow to create a sharp, lifted, cocky look.

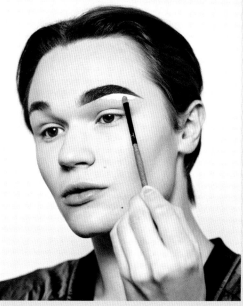

EYELINER

A little line over the eyelid . . . still, many have difficulty getting it right. Eyeliner is really tricky and requires different techniques, depending on what your eye shape is and what you want it to look like when it's done.

You know how it is: You stand in front of the mirror, so uncomfortably close that you can examine your pores, and draw the first line. You fill in the line and only want to sharpen the line a little when your hand accidentally slips. What goes through your head now is that the smallest attempt to correct the eyeliner will make it smear, so that's not possible, which leaves only one alternative, to make the line thicker. You look deeply into your eyes and say that it will be ok. The line will only get a little thicker . . . "what's the worst that could happen?" you'll remember that you said to yourself later when you're looking into the eyes of a living human panda.

I am absolutely no professional, but in this chapter I plan to go through three different eyeliners, both for hooded and nonhooded eyes.

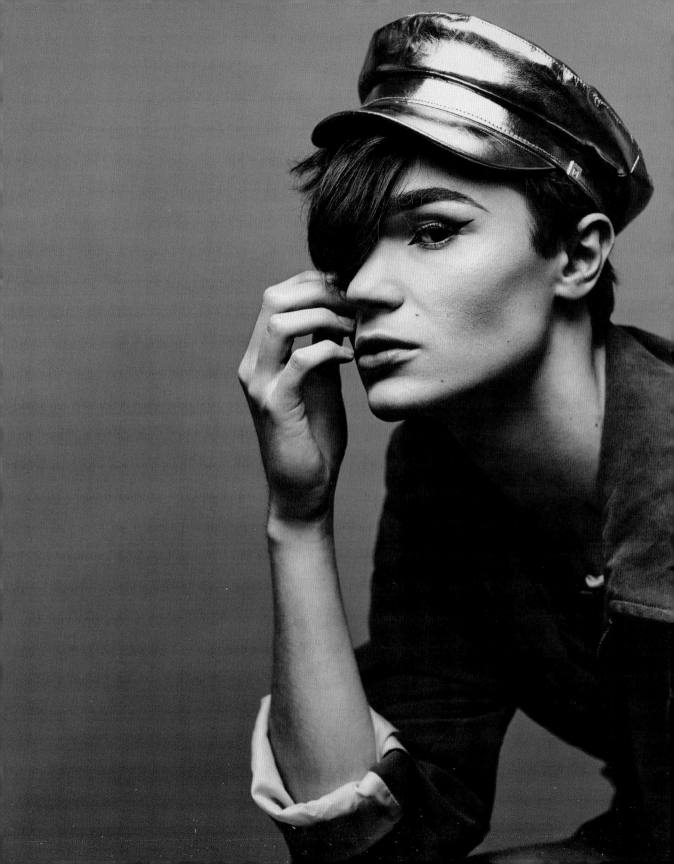

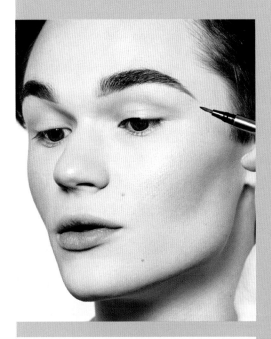

Tightlining deluxe

A thin line over the eyelid can do an incredible amount for a makeup look. Even though it is barely visible, it makes the false lashes blend in like a dream. This is the first of three different eyeliners. Classical tightlining is actually applying a kohl pencil on the upper waterline. Here I go a little farther.

STEP 1

I draw a thin line along the lash line, without making a wing. Remember to tilt the tip and almost dab the eyeliner so that it comes really close, preferably on the roots of the lashes.

STEP 2

Now I can either put on mascara and be finished or apply false lashes and mascara. I prefer to put on lashes because tightlining without anything else can make small eyes look even smaller.

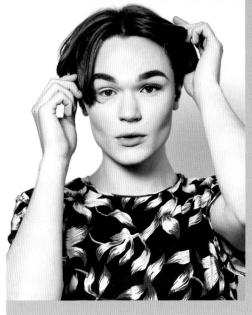

Tips!

Rest your elbow against a surface for a less shaky application.

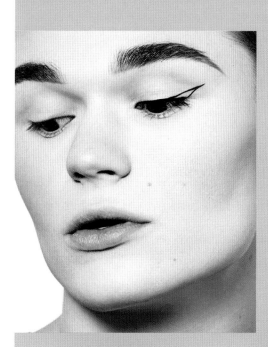

Winged

Eyeliner with wings can save many un-successfully eye makeup looks. The most important thing is not to tense your face in any way when putting it on because the result will look different when you relax. We all want the wing to be just as good looking when we take a well-planned selfie to show off, as when we're seriously staring the boss in the eyes and telling a white lie about why we can't work late.

STEP 1
Instead of settling for a thin line across the eye, I extend it. I start with the lower line in the outer corner of the eye and follow the same angle as the lower waterline.
I'll draw the upper line from the outside toward the middle of the eye. Apply the eyeliner with a little pressure to get a sharp line right away.

STEP 2
At the end, I fill in my eyeliner wing. The easiest way is to dab in the color, that way you'll have the most control.

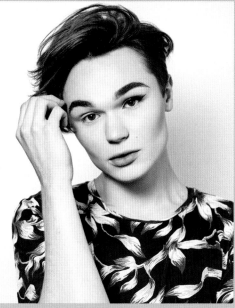

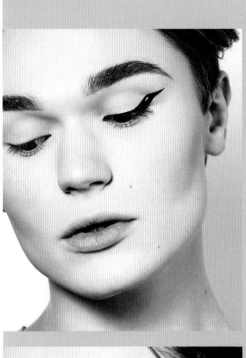

Hooded eyes

This is a trick so that hooded eyelids can wear thick eyeliner without breaking at the fold. This technique also works for a thin line.

STEP 1
I have now made a winged shape. And instead of drawing a straight line on the top of the wing, I angle it. The angle should be placed where your eyelid folds.

STEP 2
I fill the wing in and clean up underneath with concealer to make it sharp, and correct any mistakes or smears. Now I'll also extend the line toward my nose and draw it back in toward the corner of my eye.

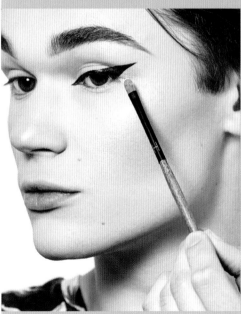

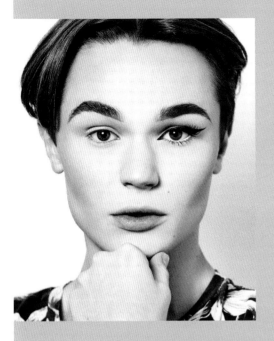

STEP 3
Here my face is relaxed and the eyeliner is
thick and fully visible, with an even shape.
Finish with a white or nude eyeliner along
the lower waterline to get a more alert
look and to give the illusion that the eye is
bigger. I tie the look together with mascara
or false lashes and mascara.

"Practice putting on eyeliner before washing off your makeup of the day."

LIPS

Lips are the icing on the cake when you have a glamorous made-up face. They tie eyebrows and eyes together and balance out the entire look.

Lip makeup has undergone significant development. In the 1920s, the lips were painted brown or plum purple. The 1940s were a fiery period for lips, and they were colored screaming red or orange. In the 1960s, the style icon Twiggy, among others, inspired the wearing of lots of lashes and light lipsticks, and in the 1980s everyone painted their lips in crazy colors, drowned them in lip gloss, and danced disco all night long.

Today, lips look quite different from even a few years ago, since liquid lipsticks, lip pencils, social media, and innovative brands and style icons have made their mark on everyday makeup.

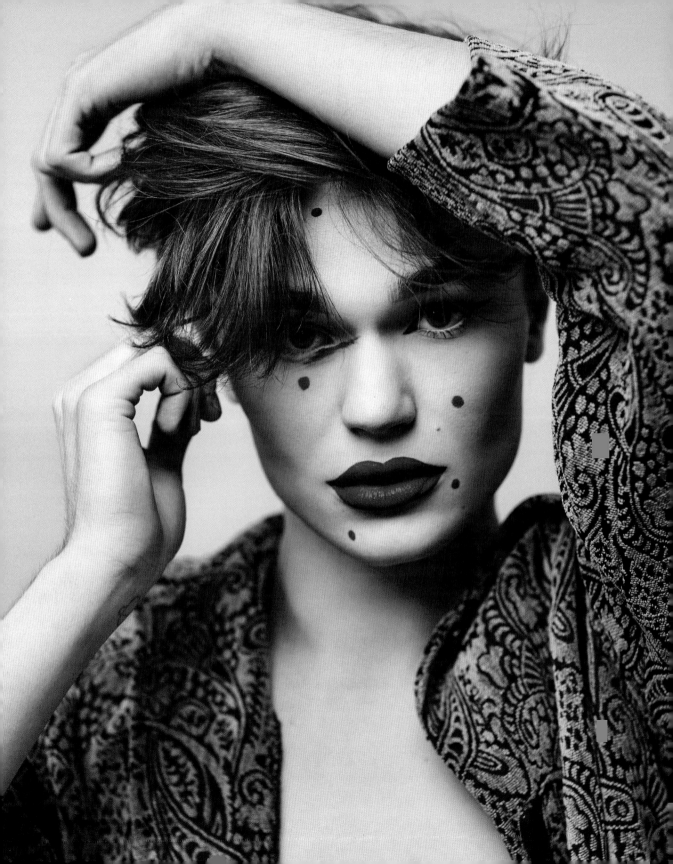

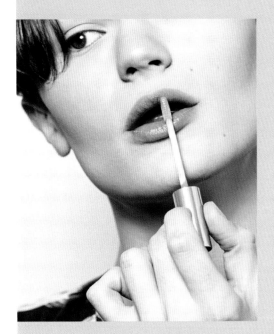

Fresh glossy

I have wide-ranging taste when it comes to makeup. I love a lot of makeup, as well as a light base with a focus on natural skin with a splash of fake freckles, simple eye makeup, and a glossy lip like this.

STEP 1

I apply the lipstick with a light hand in the middle of the lips and then spread it out either by smacking the lips against each other or by using my finger. I finish with a transparent or slightly toned lip gloss over both lips. There's only a hint of lipstick; it's the gloss that makes this mouth so spectacular.

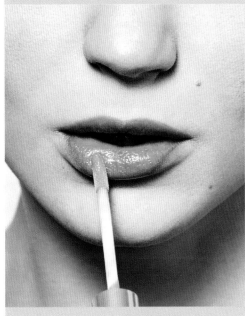

Tips!

If you want natural lips without products, gently remove the foundation from your lips using cotton swabs as if you were putting on lipstick. The color of the lips comes out; they get a certain contour, but they aren't intrusive or attention grabbing.

"A little contour shadow just below the lower lip makes the mouth poutier."

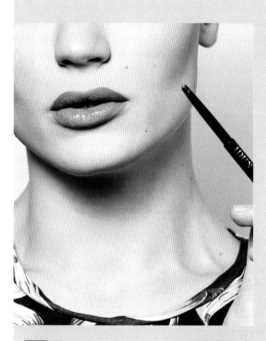

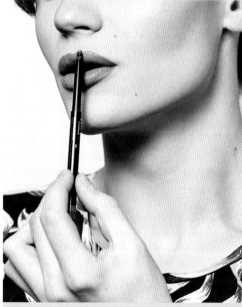

Pouty mouth

This style is just as adaptable as the eyebrows I usually create. It's perfect for a natural look if I want to have slightly fuller lips, but it also works for a heavy smokey eye as a complement to something dramatic. Creating fuller lips requires a certain technique (unless you want to look like I did when I tried my mother's red lipstick as a ten-year-old).

STEP 1

The lip liner. I start at the corners of the mouth but follow my natural lip line, and the closer to the Cupid's bow I get, the more outside of my natural lip line I go. Here, the lip liner is the mouth's equivalent to the contour shadows of the face.

STEP 2

The lines meet at Cupid's bow, and a new lip shape is created. So I follow my natural lip shape, but a few millimeters outside, but in the corners of the mouth, I keep it natural. I do the same thing on the lower lip.

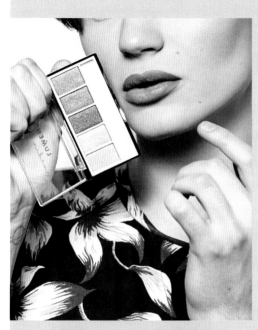

STEP 3

I smack my lips so that the lip liner blends into the middle and dab a little shimmery eye shadow on the middle of my lower lip. You can skip the eye shadow, but it gives an extra pout and a nice ombré effect.

STEP 4

Finally, I want my lips to shine and finish with a transparent lip gloss that also enhances the pout.

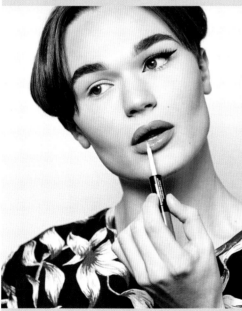

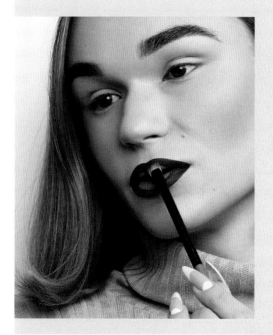

Dramatic

This third and final mouth look is of a more dramatic sort, but do not be afraid of a little color and drama; it is not as difficult as you think. Liquid matte lipstick is best for dark lips; it stays in place and can even withstand a kiss or two, if you skip the lip gloss.

STEP 1

For this particular lip, I decided to use a lip brush for more precision and control over the amount of product being used. The first step is the hardest - doing the outline. I saturate my brush in lipstick, say a prayer and start painting it on, little by little, starting at the cupid's bow. You could start at the corner of your mouth as well, but I've come to realise that this technique works best for me.

STEP 2

I leave the centre of my lips bare, and move on to a slightly brighter lip color for an ombre effect that I blend out with my ring finger. This gives the lips some dimension, but you could just fill everything in in step 1.

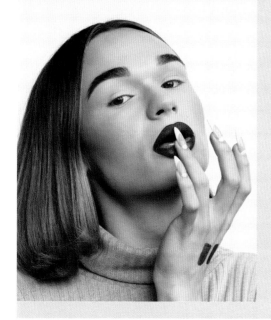

Tips!

If you combine two lipsticks, it's easiest if the colors are similar.

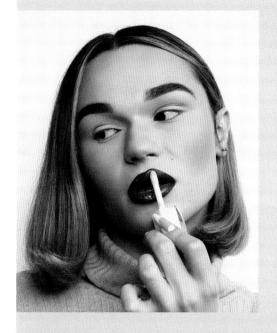

STEP 3

Gloss is love, gloss is life, right? To make
the lips a bit more juicy looking and pouty,
I top everything off with a shimmering lips
gloss. This is also optional.

*"Matte liquid lipstick is the best when
it comes to dark lips; it stays in place
and can even withstand a kiss or two, if
you skip the lip gloss."*

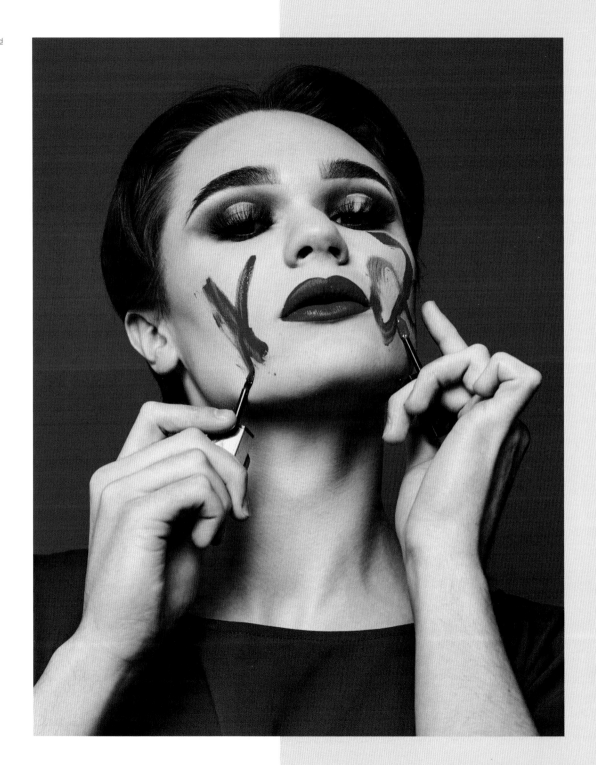

YouTube

On June 1, 2015, I published my first YouTube clip. I started with some half-nervous greetings and then introduced myself. I explained that the reason I pressed the little red recording button was that the commenters on my blog had asked for moving pictures.

I continued with a serious look saying, "We live in 2015, and I don't think that makeup defines gender, sexuality, or anything in between." And although my eye shadow in that video looks like an overambitious attempt at a smoky eye, I still stand by what I said there and then.

Most of us humans have some sort of sexuality. Gender, unlike sex organs, is a person's perception of their gender and has no actual connection to their biological sex. Norm-breaking behavior or style is not something you set out to do; it just happens the older you become and the better you get to know yourself. But it's often a reason for bullying, assault, and, in the worst cases, murder.

I don't enjoy mockery and hostility; I fight for the right and the feeling that I can be myself rather than being someone I'm not. Many LGBTQ people do not fit the stereotypes at all and get comments like "Oh, you don't seem gay." I dream of a world where sexual orientation, gender identity, ethnicity, or body shape aren't reasons to judge a person. Express your interests, accept your surroundings, let yourself and your fellow human beings rejoice and live their best possible lives.

YouTube is a platform for me to express myself, and gives an outlet for my creative side. It brings me in contact with an audience I never thought I would find. An audience that supports, encourages, and stands up for both me and each other; and who listen and respond with nuanced answers when I am in tears talking about the hard times in my life, or when I come out with the book you hold in your hands right now.

I have a lot of memories that can warm my whole body with love and joy. One of those was the first YouTube-related event in my life with about 7,000 subscribers to my channel. I was met by people who praised me for my videos and asked to take a picture with me.

Time went by, the channel grew, and I had reached 60,000 subscribers. I had my first "meet and greet," which meant that I met, took pictures, and hung out with people who wanted to meet me. My stomach contracted with nervousness before the large metal door backstage at The Stockholm Fair opened and I was surrounded by a queue of people. I stood in the booth with my friend who is also a Youtuber, and started hugging, talking, taking good-looking, funny, and silly pictures with people. Soon, two girls in their teens approached, holding each other's hands and looking nervous. They looked me in the eyes and said that my presence online as an advocate for same-sex relationships and discussions of societal problems influenced them so much that they found the strength and courage to come out to their parents about their relationship.

This makeup represents the YouTube red color, my internal flame wanting to influence and change the world, and destroy the boundaries for what is male and female.

LOOKS

I see my face as an artist sees their canvas when I am going to start making myself up. A blank canvas that can carry whatever I choose to apply, and however I choose to do it. A makeup look is my equivalent to a finished painting.

A pink eye shadow can be my shade for an artistic look, and a painted glitter tear from my eye can represent my grief. With makeup it's possible to convey a thousand words without saying a single one. In this chapter I will go through a number of different looks that hopefully will inspire, teach, or challenge you. Spread out your makeup in front of your makeup mirror or fill up the sink if you do your makeup in the bathroom, put on the artist smock, and start splashing, dabbing, or swiping all the colors in the color wheel on your face!

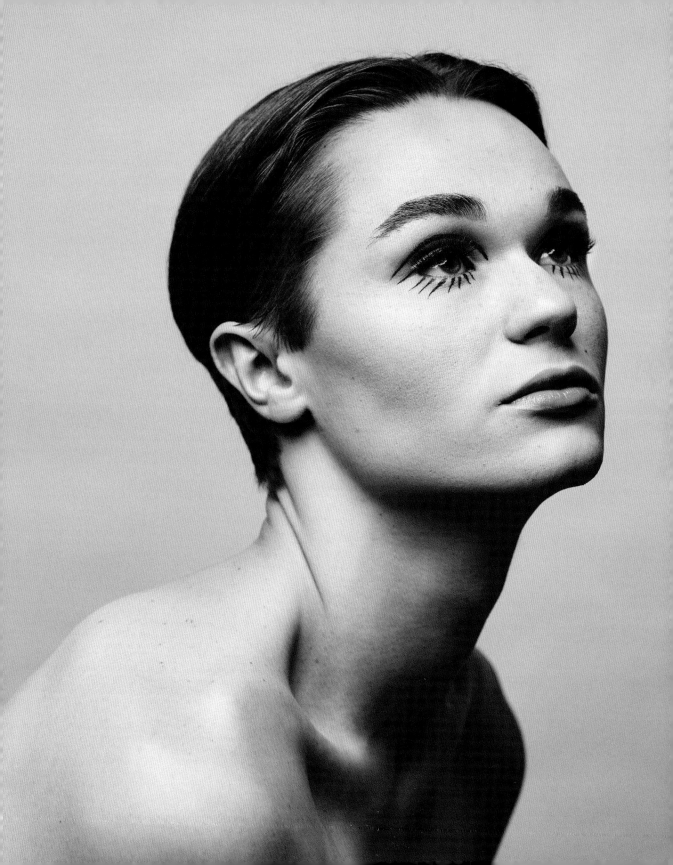

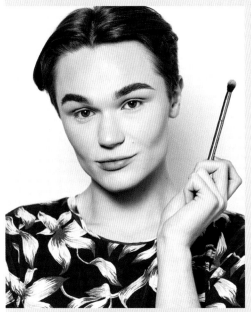

Natural

A fresh and light makeup look with a focus on skin and brows.

STEP 1
I start by applying a thin layer of liquid foundation, mixed with a liquid highlighter on my face, and dab on a cream blush. I keep the contouring very light and sweep a little bronzer over my cheeks, forehead, and nose. The contour palette I also use as an eye shadow palette. I draw on a pair of full but very natural brows.

STEP 2
Now I apply lip gloss, a little mascara, and finally a little setting spray so that the foundation and powder melts together and the highlights appear.

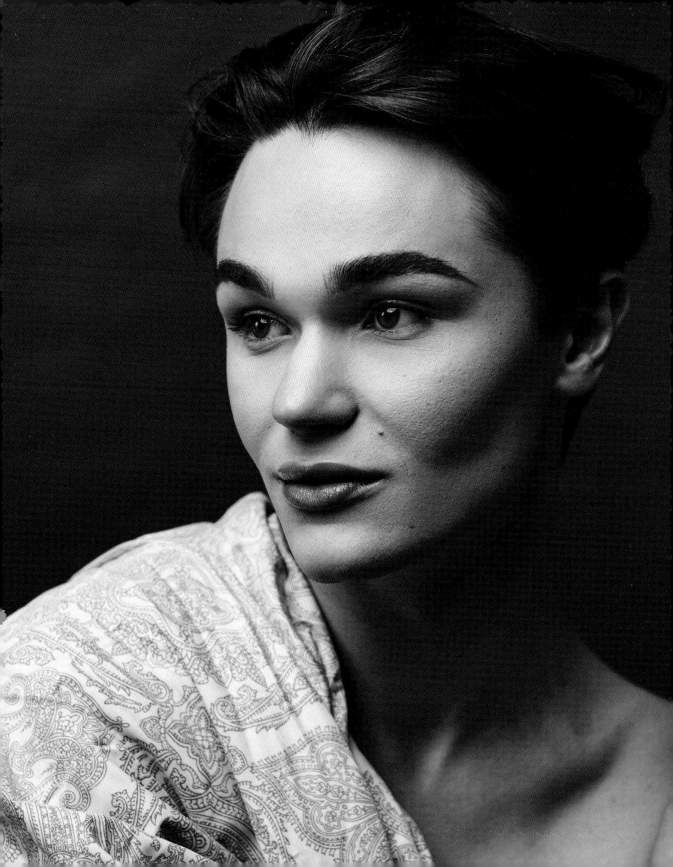

Kardashian wet look

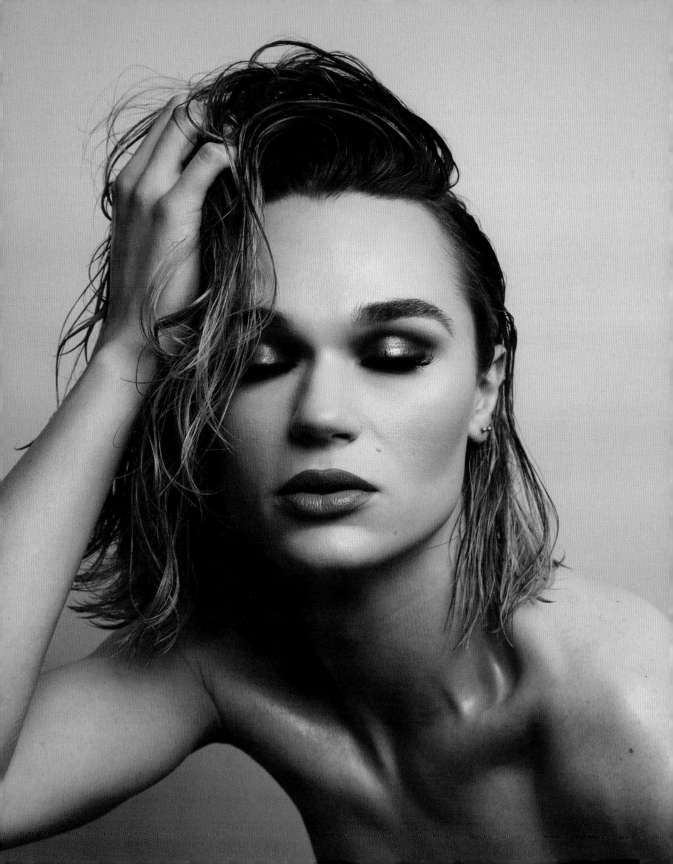

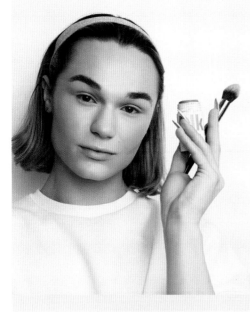

Kim Kardashian wet look

Kim Kardashian is a woman who, with her makeup artist Mario Dedivanovic, influenced many in the makeup world. For many years, these two have been associated with a look with a classic heavier contouring that contrasts with bright areas under the eyes, in the middle of the forehead, along the nose, and on the chin, baked with thick layers of powder. This is my take on Mario and Kim's iconic wet MET gala look which I really don't think is a dunk-your-face-in-powder type of look. Hear me out, I'll go through it.

STEP 1

I use a concealer that is 2 shades lighter than my foundation for a highlighted look. To sculpt the face I use a contour/bronzer stick that I stipple on with a brush. I like this technique rather than drawing lines on my face with the stick because I have more control over the amount of product and it is easier to blend out. I only fully set my under eye concealer, the rest of the face is just lightly dusted to still have a bit of sheen. I mean, we are after all doing a really dewy look.

STEP 2

For the transition shade in my crease I use a warm brown eyeshadow that I blend out with a fluffy brush and then start packing on a burgundy brown shade with a flat brush in the inner and outer corners of my eye.

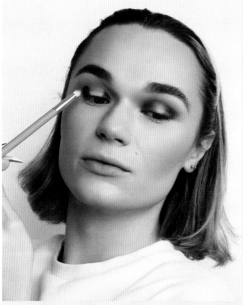

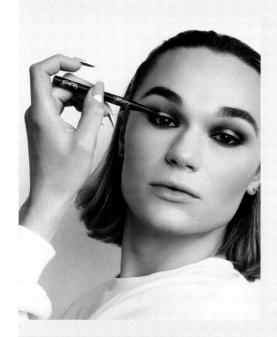

I then begin to go over the edges of the burgundy shade with a small detailing brush to blend it out. Take your time, this part can be tricky. Leave the centre of the lid bare.

STEP 3

Closest to the lower lash line I apply a black shadow, that I then blend lower down with the burgundy and finish it off by touching up the edges with the warm brown shade for a smooth transition from dark to warm brown. Along the upper lashes, I apply a thin eyeliner.

STEP 4

To really get the glow going, I cover the bare part of my eyelid with a shimmering eyeshadow with glitter specs in it. For the lips there is no other option than nude, so I pair a darker liquid lipstick, with a lighter lipgloss for some definition. I drench my chest and shoulders in a body oil and use an eye cream on my cheekbones, nose and chin on top of my powder highlight for a skinlike, ultra glowing finish.

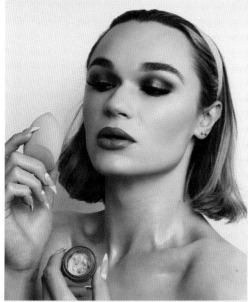

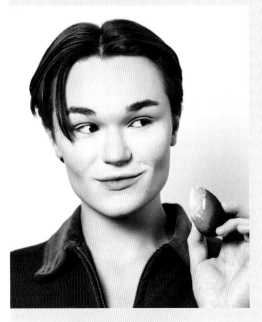

Day

If you're leaving home in the morning, knowing you won't have time to redo, only touch up, your makeup before heading to the club, here's some tips and tricks for your makeup to stay intact both day and night.

STEP 1
For me, a long-lasting, nice stylish base goes hand in hand with powder. I start by baking my base a little extra, since I have tonight's escapades in mind.

STEP 2
I contour my face lightly, put a little brow gel in my eyebrows so that they stay in place during the day.

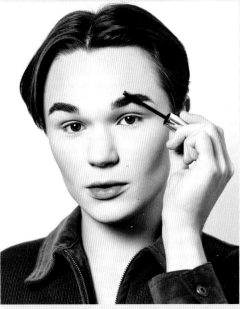

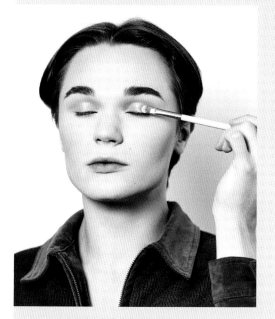

STEP 3
Last but not least, I shade the crease with my contour palette and apply the same highlighter to my eyelids that I used on my face.

"The more mature your skin, the fewer powder products you should use."

Day

Night

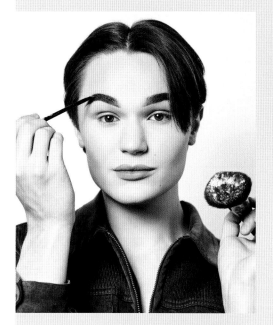

Night

If you want to spice your day-look up but don't have the time to do it from scratch, I'm here to guide you through the stress.

STEP 1
I powder the areas that got shiny during the day, fill in my eyebrows to the desired shape and intensity, and contour my face a little more.

STEP 2
I make the earthy tones I've had on my eyes to this point more red-toned with eye shadows that I build up from light to dark.

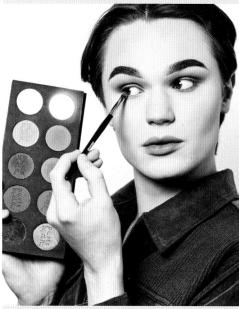

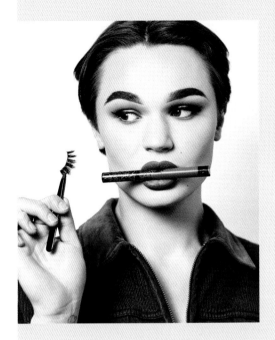

STEP 3

Finally, I apply a pair of false lashes and apply lipstick. I stick to the same color scale as the eye shadow.

Blue

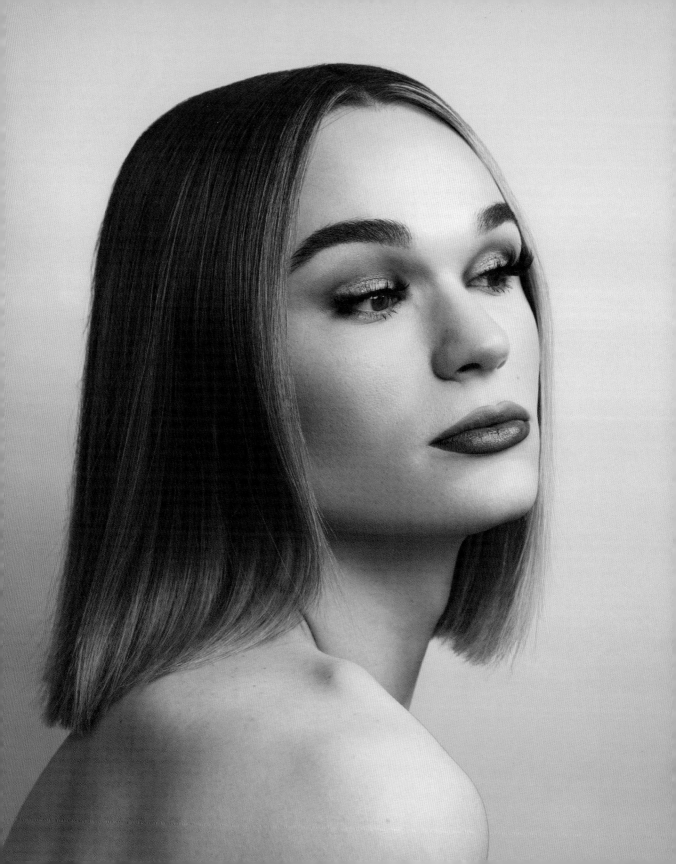

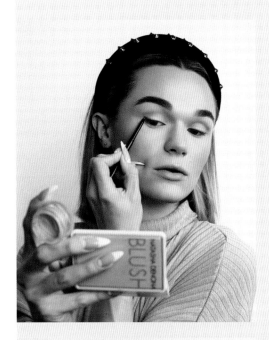

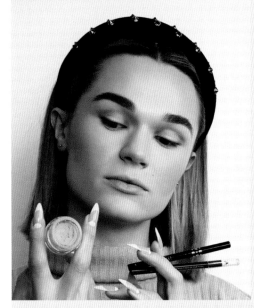

Blue

Sometimes I put myself in front of my makeup mirror and feel the need to take my overflowing glass of creativity and pour it all over myself. It often results in me starting to do my makeup, trying new techniques, and hearing how all my colorful palettes sing a seductive choral song that makes me set aside all my plans for a natural eye look.

STEP 1

A trick for getting better color payoff when doing colorful looks is to do a base to the eyeshadow with a pencil or cream product. It gives the eyeshadow something to stick to and the risk of it being patchy is smaller. Here I define my crease with a light blue cream color and darken my outer corner with an eye pencil in a darker blue tone for depth. This is blended out with a small detailing brush.

STEP 2

Using an even deeper blue, I darken the outer corner of my lid. I do the same with my inner corner and lower lashline, leaving the middle-most part bare, both on the lid and under the eye. The closer I get to either the inner or outer corner, the deeper the blue shade.

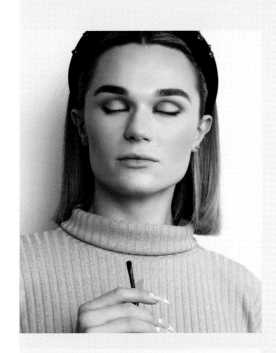

STEP 3

With two tones of blue eyeshadow, I set the pencil and cream products with the same technique and blend them out seamlessly with a small detailing brush in tiny, circular motions. Remember to keep it the darkest in both corners and softly blending them into the crease for a defined look.

STEP 4

I mix loose glitter with a mixing liquid and apply this onto the bare areas on my lid and the lower lashline, pop on a pair of lashes and fill my lips in with the two pencils. The darker one does on the bottom lip, and the lighter one on the upper. This is topped off with a sparkling gloss. If you'd like to keep the look a bit more toned down, go for a nude color.

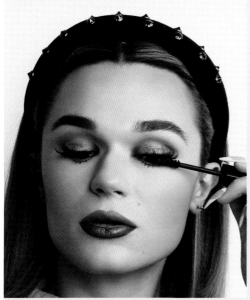

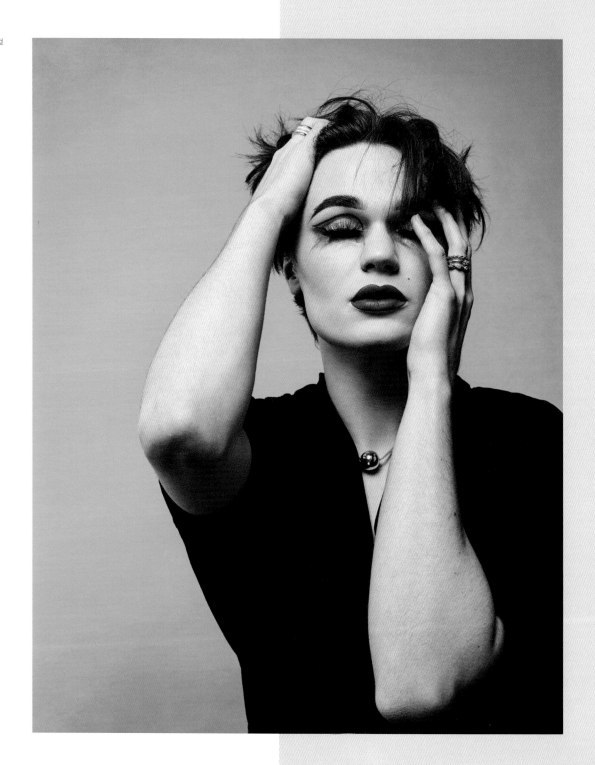

ADHD

The year before I graduated from high school, I was diagnosed with attention deficit hyperactivity disorder (ADHD). ADHD is a neuropsychiatric spectrum disorder that is mainly linked to hyperactivity, impulsivity, and difficulty concentrating. A common misconception about people with ADHD is that they are aggressive, constantly disturbing and annoying the people around them.

In school, I was in a very accepting and friendly class that never pointed out my ADHD, but I never wanted to ask for accommodations at school, like having a separate room to be able to concentrate on a task. I did not want to feel different or be a burden to the teacher or my classmates, but when I think of that time, I wish I had prioritized my own condition more. The older you get, the better you know yourself, your routines, and your needs. I work best in a quiet room without distractions and have a hard time sitting in a room of mumbling people with six conversations going on at the same time. I respond to the classic question: What advice would you give to your younger self? I would say that he should realize that his so-called condition would resolve itself when he finds an outlet where he can channel his hyperactivity and need for creative stimulation. But before he finds that outlet, he has to reach out and get some help along the way, and recognize the obvious choice between being able to concentrate or intentionally making school more difficult.

When I got my diagnosis, they immediately offered me medication and I said yes because I thought it was necessary for a fully functioning life, but that wasn't the case I realized later. I tried different medications that all involved changing activity in certain areas of the brain, for example improving the ability to pay attention, the ability to concentrate, and to reduce impulsivity.

I felt quite apathetic, as my joy was not particularly joyful and my lows were not stressful in any way, which made everyday life very monotonous and gray. Medication is very individual, and sometimes is the solution to the problems that can arise in everyday life. For me, it's better without medication because I found my focus at the same time as I found YouTube. When I realized that I could devote all my excess energy and creativity to my new interest, the balance in my life got much better. I was back to having peaks and valleys, but I prefer feeling this way, to being as we say in Sweden, *lagom*, that is, moderate or just enough all the time.

My ADHD isn't an impairment; this look is my creativity personified, right here, right now. My ADHD is a power that helps me to do what I do best, a little better and a little more. When my brain starts going, there is no way out except to find an outlet for my creativity.

Twiggy

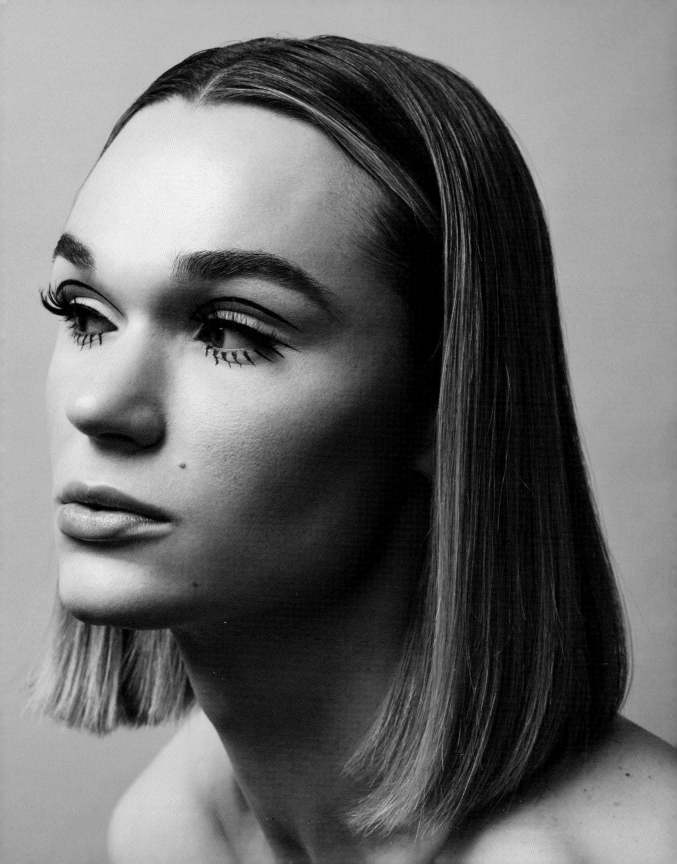

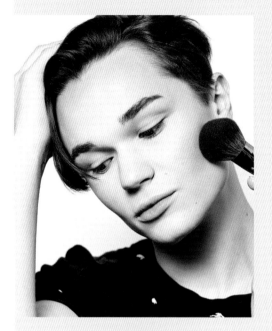

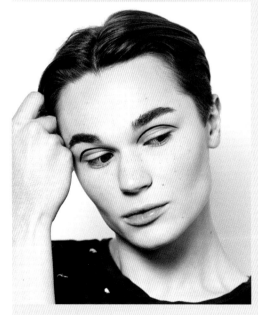

Twiggy

The makeup trends of the 1950s were based on pastel colors, minimal contouring, with a lot of focus on the lips. A decade later, interest moved to the eyes, eyes, and only eyes. Neither the face nor the lips were in focus, and false eyelashes started being used every day to enlarge and mark the eyes. The style and makeup icon Twiggy created a special, graphic, and very unique look.

STEP 1

Twiggy didn't have coverage as top priority. Powder, on the other hand, was everyone's best friend in the 1960s. Here I keep the base very natural by applying a little foundation and working it in all over the whole face. Then I matte it down with a powder.

STEP 2

I drag my eyebrow pencil lightly through my brows and put gel on them to avoid a dusty appearance from all the powder. With the same pencil I also make freckles on and around my nose. Here I do not use the "splash method" (see page 98), because I only want a few freckles. I mattify my eyelids with a bone white shadow and draw a line above my natural crease with a gel liner and a thin eyeliner brush, so that it's visible when my eyes are open, then blend it out a little.

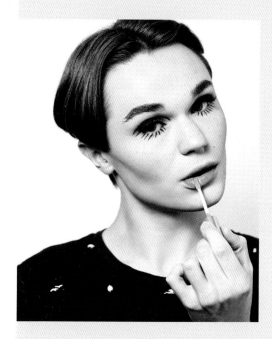

STEP 3

Then I take my eyeliner pen and draw a thin line on my eyelid to allow my false lashes to melt in seamlessly. Finally, I draw lash-like lines under the lower lash line for a doll-like look.

"The style and makeup icon Twiggy created a special, graphic, and very unique look."

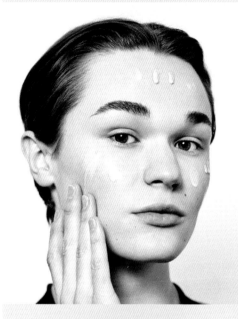

Glow

There is glow, and then there is *glow*. The best base for me is the one that looks better three hours after you put it on because the foundation, the liquid highlights, and the powder you fixed everything with have melted together and look like skin, not makeup. I have touched on the subject before, but I'm coming back to the inner glow some people get when they're pregnant. I love this look and it can definitely be said that I'm aiming for the pregnancy glow when I put makeup on. I would also like to urge anyone who confuses glow with oiliness to try this light and fresh makeup look.

STEP 1
The glow starts already during my foundation with a liquid highlighter on the highest points of my face. This ensures that the highest points will get extra glow when everything melts together.

STEP 2
I also mix my foundation with a few drops of liquid highlighter. So my face will have a slight glow, while the highest points that also have liquid highlighter underneath them will get extra glow during the day when the products have fused with the natural oils from my skin.

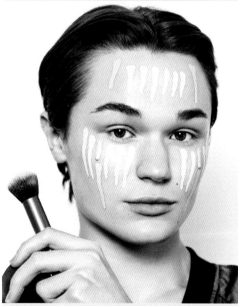

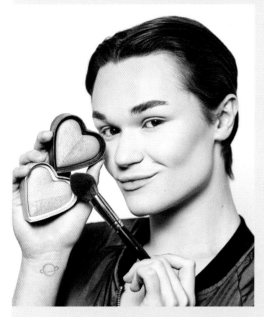

STEP 3

When I do makeup with glow, I naturally focus on the shimmering products. I apply a light shading for a natural look and reinforce my facial structure with a warmer, shimmery powder that I then blend together with a blush. It is easy to overdo it here and become too orange; therefore I recommend doing this step in natural light or at least in light that is not too yellow.

STEP 4

My eyebrows are painted, and then I move on to the eye shadow. With circular and back-and-forth motions, I build up a transition color with only warm colors. The lightest color is applied to the largest area, meaning that I blend this almost up to the eyebrow. The darker the color you apply, the smaller the surface and closer to the crease it should be.

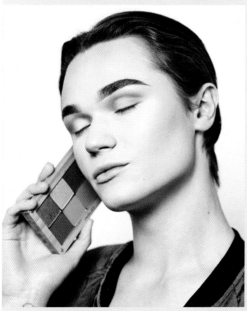

Tips!

Blend your highlighter into your shimmering blush and bronzer instead of applying it to a matte base to build up an intense but natural glow.

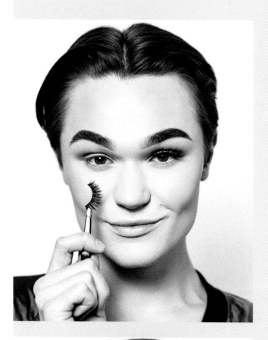

STEP 5

On my eyelid I put a liquid eye shadow with a lot of shimmer that dries. It is much like a liquid lipstick, with shimmer, but for the eyes! I put a little more orange in the outer edge of the eyelid, make the same color combination along the lower lash line, and tie the top and bottom together. Finally, I apply a pair of false lashes and put white eyeliner on my waterline.

STEP 6

To complete the look, I apply liquid lipstick and, on top of it, a transparent lip gloss.

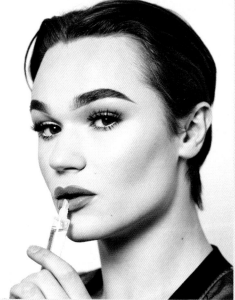

Tips!

A transparent lip gloss makes all matte lipstick shiny without changing the color

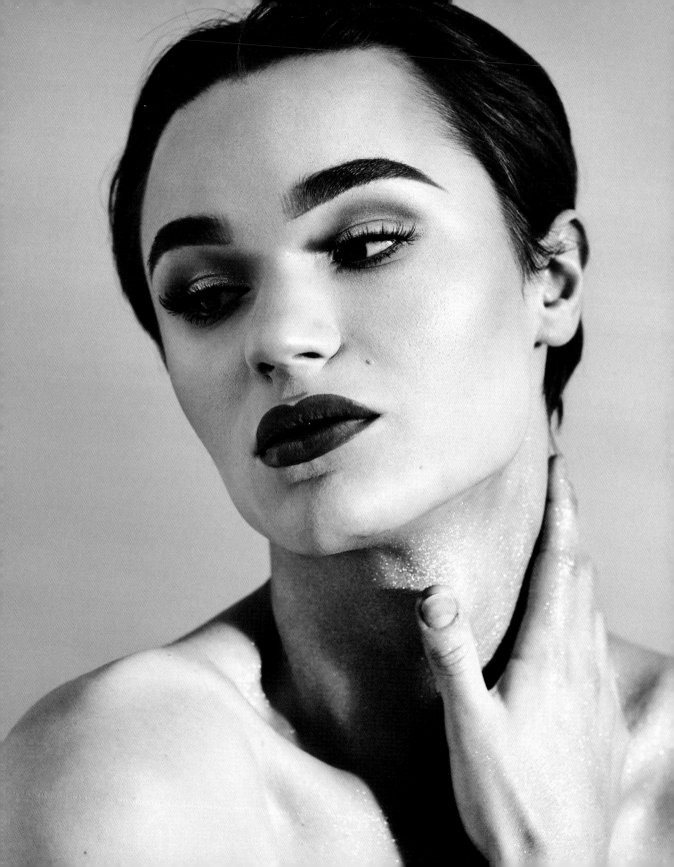

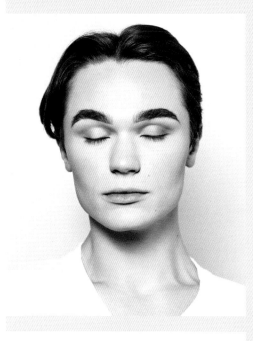

Cheap vs. expensive

We have all asked ourselves if you really need to put hundreds of dollars into a palette when there are cheaper alternatives. Can't we settle for a palette that isn't the same price as a mortgage on a Manhattan apartment?

There are many reasons why two palettes with similar shades can have drastically differing prices. It's about ingredients, packaging, quality, and the brand's status, to name a few. But often cheap doesn't mean bad. Here I make up my eyes with each palette to compare them. The half face on the right of the pictures is made up with the expensive palette, and the one on the left with the cheaper one.

STEP 1

With the brown, matte shadows in the palettes, I build up a shadow in the crease and on my outer V. I do not notice much difference in how easy the different shadows are to blend, but the pigmentation is better on the expensive side. Some eye shadows tend not to want to be moved from where they first touched your skin, but these all blended out without any problems.

STEP 2

I switch to chocolate-brown shadows and continue my earth toned theme to darken the makeup from the center of the eyelid to the outer edge. I notice that the darker the shadows I use, the weaker the pigmentation of the cheap side, but the shadow still blends out very easily. It is possible to build up the color, but after packing too much eye shadow, it becomes more difficult to blend out. The expensive side has good pigmentation, which is not difficult to blend out but has a bit too much fallout when dipping the brush into the product.

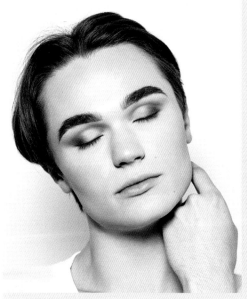

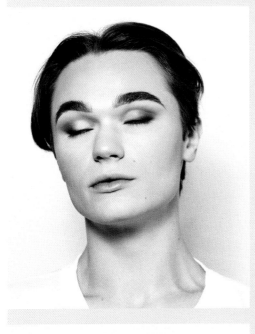

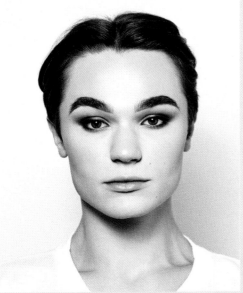

STEP 3

Here I apply a golden shimmer shadow on each eyelid and slightly blend it into the transition color on my crease. Next, I smoke up the makeup by applying a faded eyeliner along the lashline. It is easiest to notice how good a palette is when applying shimmer shadows and the palette's black shadow. On the expensive side, I get the result I want from the shimmer; I don't fall off the chair in absolute shock but I'm happy with the result. The black shade has good pigmentation and does not turn out to be dull when blended, but the blending itself could have been easier for such an expensive palette. The cheap palette did not do what I wanted. The shimmer was too powdery, which resulted in a lot of product falling off the eyelid. The black shadow was buildable, to some extent, but didn't equal the expensive palette's pigmentation.

STEP 4

Finally, I do the same combination under the lower lash line. From the outer corner in, I put black, dark and lighter brown, and a golden shimmer at the inner corner.

The result of the comparison is that the cheap palette, for its price, isn't bad, and that the expensive palette lived up to my expectations but still is a bit expensive. If you have a few extra twenties every month and really want this particular palette, I don't think you should hesitate; it is a good palette. If you don't have a palette, I advise you to buy two for the price of one of these. Palettes with a price tag of around $25-30 USD can be very good, and you get a greater variety of colors.

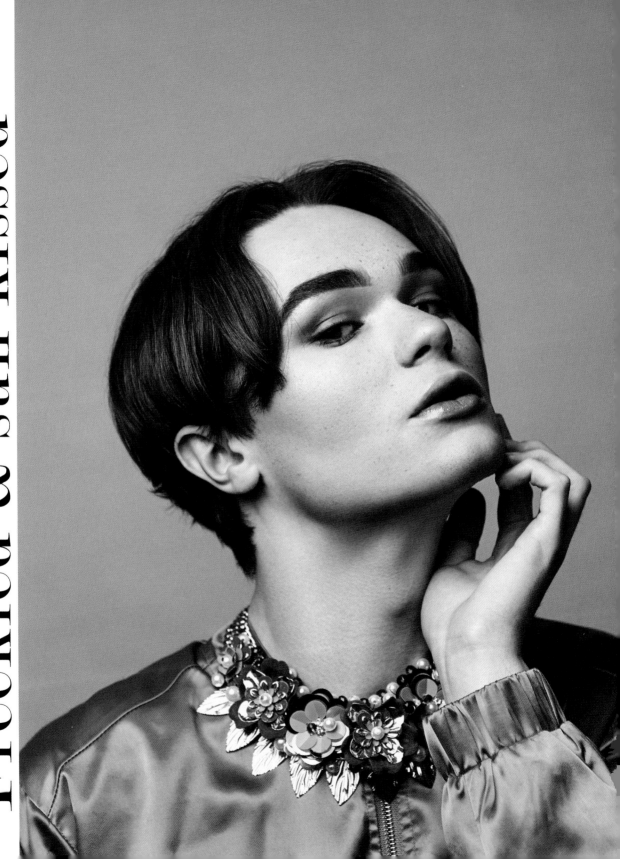

Freckled & sun kissed

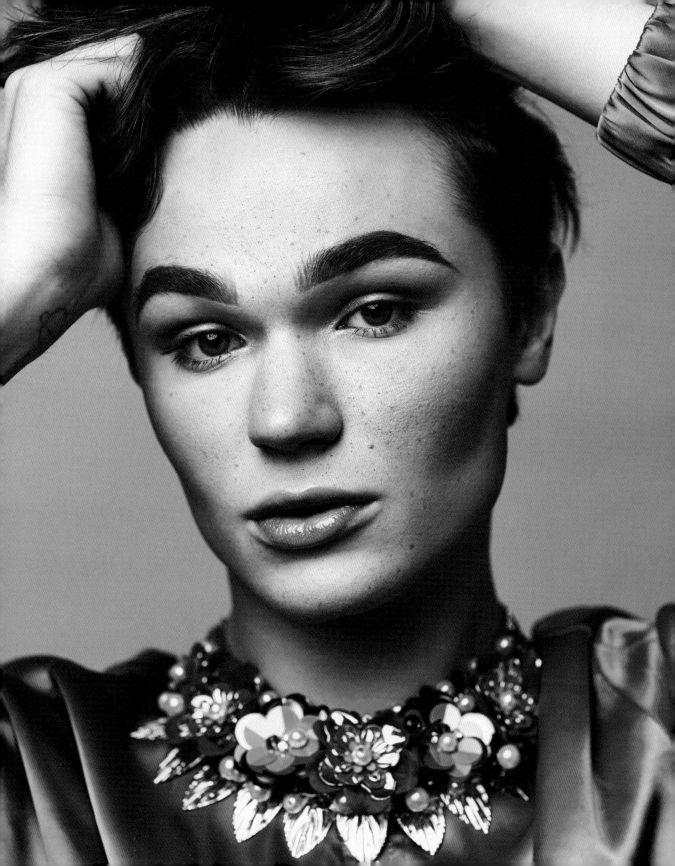

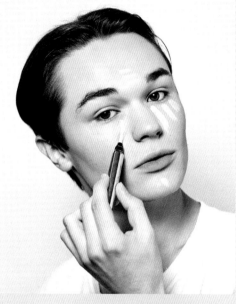

Freckled & sun kissed

When I sunbathe, whether abroad or in Sweden, I get a nice sun-kissed look, especially on my face. Some parts of my face become a little more tan than others because of where the sun hits it, my green-brown eyes become greener, and my glow becomes very prominent. Makeup is, in my opinion, a form of art, and in the following makeup I am Leonardo da Vinci, my face is my canvas, you are my apprentice, and I will teach you how to paint a freckled, sun-kissed face.

STEP 1

I apply a very light base with foundation and then a very light concealer. I want to give the impression that my sun-kissed face is genuine, not made-up; so I keep the base minimal so that the skin can shine through.

STEP 2

I keep the contouring to a minimum and instead pour on bronzer in volume. Cheeks, forehead, and nose are the most important. I apply the bronzer straight across my nose instead of along it; it increases the sun-kissed impression.

STEP 3

Freckles! I pour some water into a powder lid and mix everything that can color the water to about the same color as my hair, whether with cocoa, coffee, or an old eye shadow—be creative! Then I take a round foundation brush, dip it lightly in the water, and then pull the thumb over the bristles so that the water will splash on my face. Try sprinkling the droplets once in the sink before splashing on your face. I continue with this until I have a base of freckles, and then make some bigger with the help of a newly sharpened eyebrow pencil.

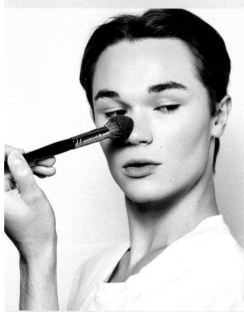

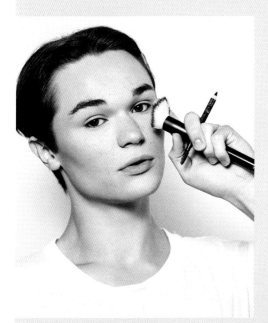

STEP 4

I fill my brows with the same eyebrow pencil and put a simple shade in the crease with warm tones.

STEP 5

I finish with a golden shimmer on my eyelid and a champagne-colored shadow in the inner corner of the eye. On my lips I add a lip gloss with multireflective glitter particles, for a glazed-donut look.

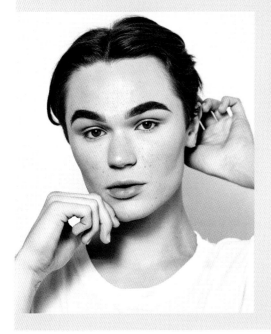

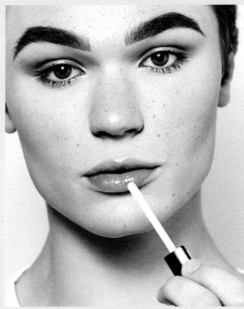

Gold

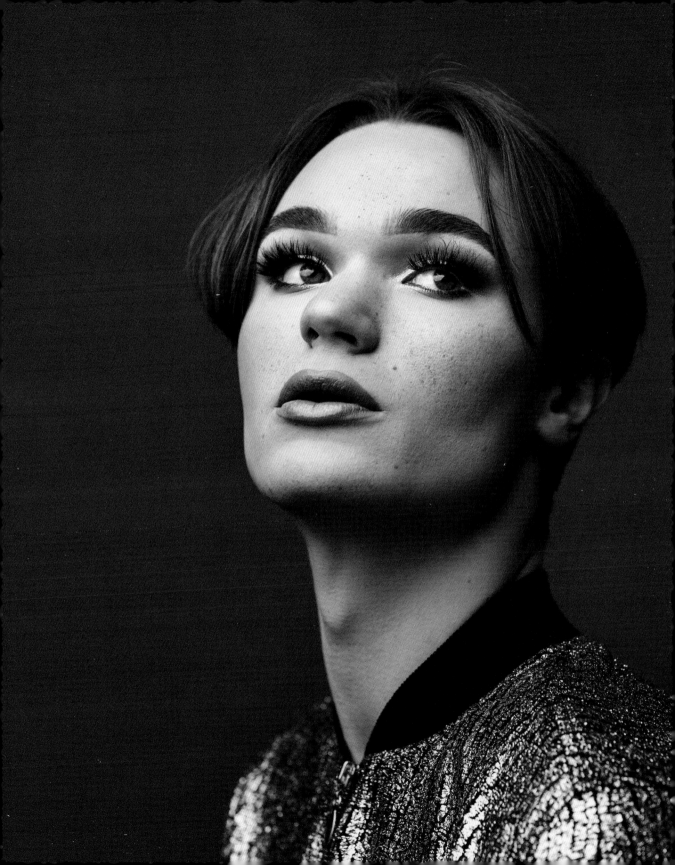

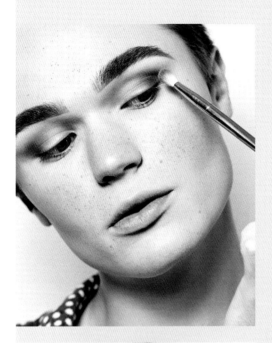

Gold

I love to have shimmer on my eyelids, not least of which is gold.

STEP 1

I first build up a transition color in the crease with a fluffy brush. I start with a light brown and then go over to a warm, darker shade that I concentrate in the outer edge of the crease and lightly sweep it in toward the inner part of the eye and blend it down on the outer edge of the eyelid. Blending it on the eyelid is not necessary, but I think the black mixes better with the brown later on if I do.

STEP 2

The theme color, gold, I'll put directly on my finger and apply in small trails over two-thirds of my eyelid and then lightly combine it with the transition color in the crease, to avoid sharp edges. Applying shimmer shadows with your finger always gives the best payoff.

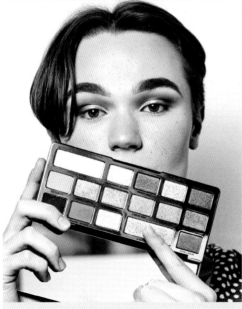

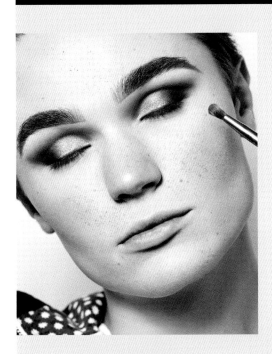

STEP 3

With a small, fluffy brush, I apply the black shade of the palette to the outer edge of my eyelid. First I pack on the shadow, then I blend out the edges. In this way I get the most intensity instead of fading the shadow. I combine the black with the crease color and also blend in the golden tone.

STEP 4

I also put the gold in the inner corner of my eye and under the lower lash line. Then I tie together the makeup with black shadow in the outer corner of my eye.

STEP 5

Finally, I apply false lashes and put two dots at the corner of the eye for a more detailed look. The lashes are fluffy and flirtatious and take the makeup from glamorous to, as Fergie sings, "g-l-a-m-o-r-o-u-s."

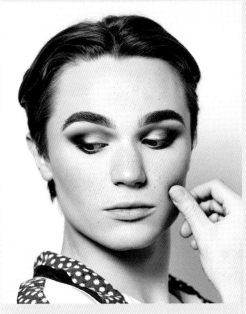

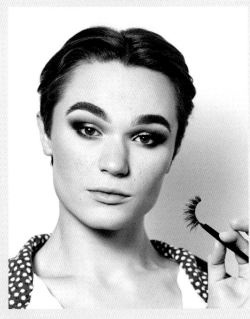

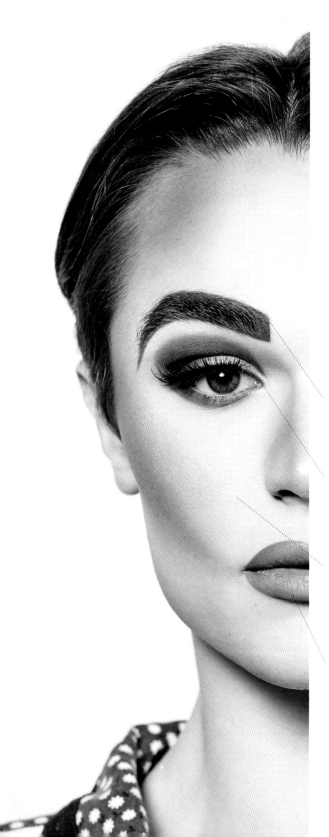

Do's & don't's

I started makeup when I was seventeen and quickly realized what I had learned by following beauty gurus on the internet was not enough for good execution in practice. I knew about how to apply a false eyelash but could not, for the life of me, attach it where I wanted it to go.

Here I go through the most-common mistakes when it comes to powder products, lips, brows, and eyes. Your makeup is again something that you should be happy with and comfortable in; this is only to help those of you who want a better result but don't know how to go about it.

Eyebrows: Boxy, too long and they give the impression that the face is drooping.

Eyes: The edges of the eye shadow are sharp and not blended, and the eyelashes are placed too far out.

Contouring: An intense shading can be amazing, but not a patchy contouring, which, on the forehead, gives the impression of a dirty face. A contour line that goes too far toward the mouth counteracts its purpose.

Lips: The overlining begins in the corners of the mouth.

Avoid

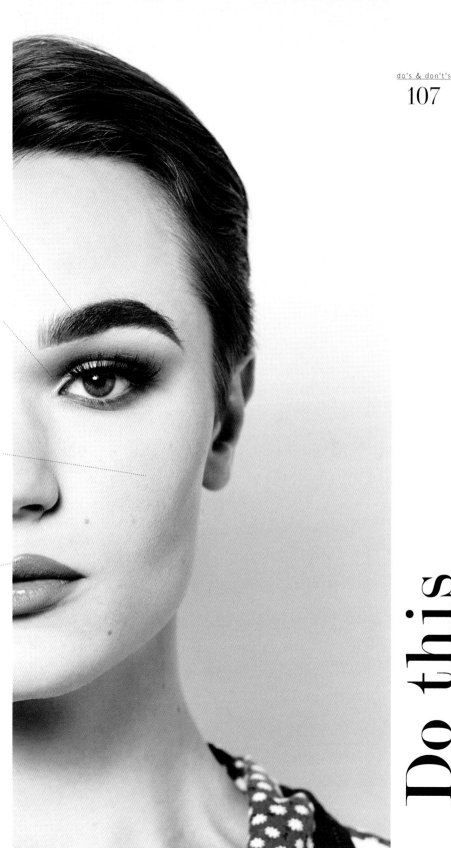

Eyebrows: Go a little lighter with the eyebrow pencil at the innermost part of the eyebrow to soften and get a more natural brow. End the tail higher up to get a lifted expression instead of creating an unnecessary drooping impression.

Eyes: Carefully blend out the eye shadow to avoid patchy areas and to create the perfect transition between colors. The false lashes should be placed as close to the eyelashes as possible and always have a few millimeters of margin to the outer corner of the eye to avoid the lash poking and the eye looking droopy.

Contouring: Build your contour color a little at a time; it's easier to add to than to remove what has already been worked into your base. Remember not to draw the line too far toward the mouth, where there are no natural shadows to enhance.

Lips: The trick is not to start overlining in the corners of the mouth. Apply outside the lipline more and more the closer to the cupid's bow you get, to get a neat pout.

Do this

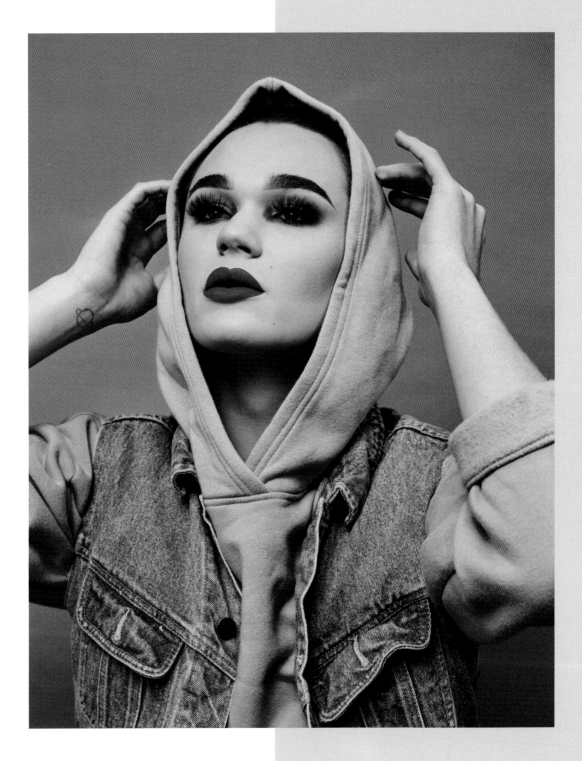

MY STORY:

Music

I was a very happy little kid. Lots of things made me laugh, like when I sat in my swing that hung from a strong beam in the ceiling, bouncing up and down on the floor, or when I went with my grandmother to the preschool and asked for three pieces of gum to blow big bubbles that in the end just got stuck all over my face.

But what really got my body bubbling over and my brain activity to shoot through the ceiling then, and still does today, is music. Creating a chord sequence with an instrument, then combining it with a melody loop that gets the listener to cry or feel the tension rising in their chest, or weep with joy, is something that fascinates me. Admittedly, I didn't think of it that way when I was small, but I was moved by all the music I heard.

I started in a children's choir, which expanded my musical horizons considerably. I moved from simply thinking that Céline Dion had a powerful singing voice to understanding about breath control, pronunciation, and articulation. In the choir, I found lyrics and voices in a completely different way than what was offered by my mother's CDs that I lip-synched to in the living room. Not long afterwards, we learned about notes and then I embraced my mom's interest in violin and wanted to learn to play. This led to lessons with the school's vocal instructor and I happily attended weekly choir, solo, orchestra, and violin lessons for four years.

When my interest in violin waned, my interest in singing continued for a few more years, until nearing the end of gymnasium, when my YouTube career took off and my interest in singing had to live on, still close to my heart, but without singing lessons.

About a year ago I started writing and singing my own music. It's opened a whole new door, helped me flourish, and made me who I am today: a music nerd who asks people at a party to be quiet because my latest favorite song has a low, kind of uniquely mixed bass line in the background that ends with a lively drum part, and I really want to hear it. I'm gripped by an inner ecstasy when good production meets a good melody, and my brain has to mix the signals for pleasure and hearing and instead think, "Pulling together both is a right in any case."

Creating, listening to, and growing through music is something I never want to stop. I can sit for hours and work without getting tired, and I am absolutely convinced that I have something unique to give the world. This makeup represents my cockiness, my humility, and my playfulness when it comes to music.

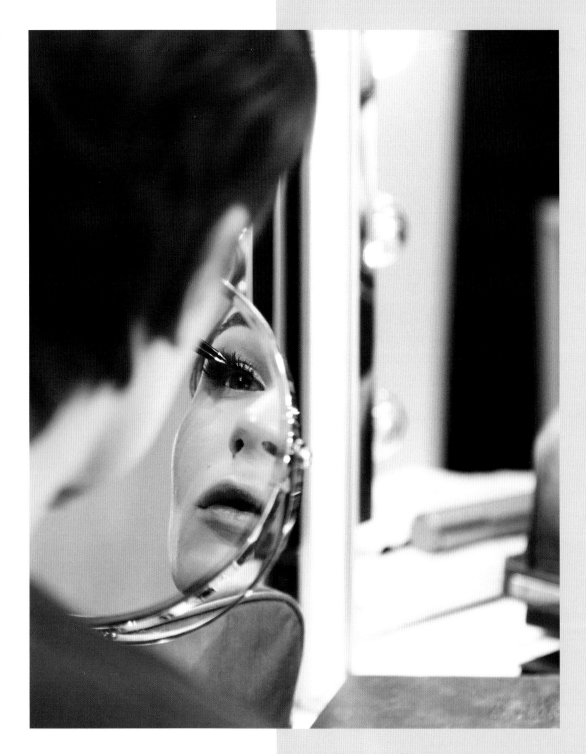

Q&A

Here I've collected questions that I often get from my followers. Many people want to know how I do my makeup, which brands I use, and what my favorite products are. Other people have questions about their own makeup. Here are your questions and my answers!

Questions about me:

How many times a day do you wash your face?
Ideally, twice. Realistically, once, in the evening. I do however do my skincare right before doing my makeup because I think it applies way better than relying on the skincare I did the night before. So to make a long answer short, I wash it once or twice a day, depending on if I do my makeup or not.

What skin type do you have?
(dry, oily, normal; combination skin)
I have combination skin, or at least I think so. My skin is usually normal, except in the T zone, which has a tendency to get oily. Whatever your skin type is, always tailor your routine having that in mind.

Do you exfoliate your skin?
Yes, once or twice a week to remove the layer of dead skin cells that a regular washing won't get rid of. I don't over exfoliate though, as that can leave my skin dry and damaged. I stick to a physical exfoliation tool with tiny silicone bristles to lightly exfoliate and help with removing any dirt/makeup, and once or twice a week I use a scrub or a chemical peeling.

Do you have or have you had problems with acne?
My skin is not prone to acne and has never been. The only problem I've had and have is actually my forehead. I get small, closed pores that I think are called closed comedones that can't be squeezed nor should they, and I can't do much about them except exfoliate or the regular. Don't give up when it comes to skin care; once you've found what works for you, only routine and willpower will yield results. It was much worse in my teenage years.

Do you know what undertone your skin has?
This can be very tricky. Your undertone is either warm (gold, yellow), cool (red, pink, blue) or neutral (olive). I've tried and tried to find it and I would place myself closer to the warm side. Two ways to determine this is to either look at the color of your veins or if you look the best in silver or gold jewelry. Green veins means warm undertone, blue means cool. Gold jewelry means warm undertone, silver means cool. You could also determine this by wrapping yourself in a white towel—apparently your undertones become more apparent.

Face care

What do you think about false eyelashes?
Love, love, love them! I was a very "the bigger the better" kind of girl, but as I've branched into different looks, I also pair it with the most fitting eyelash—some tickling my eyebrows, some just adding a wispy flair.

What makeup tools do you use to apply makeup?
I would say most of them. I love to have a bundle of brushes in front of me and be able to pick and choose as I want. A must in my makeup bag, however, is a makeup sponge to get my desired finish from my base products.

Do you use primer before applying eye makeup?
No, I actually don't. Why, I don't know; I just never needed it since my eyelids didn't tend to get oily and make my eye shadow crease. But I use something that behaves almost like an eye shadow primer, concealer!

What is your favorite eye shadow (color)?
I am absolutely in love with all kinds of warm shadows like orange and red. She's basic, but can you blame her? A good sunset eye look, I mean come on!

What do you think of drugstore makeup?
For me, it doesn't matter if my makeup is expensive or cheap; if it performs well, I'm satisfied.

Have you thought about learning from a professional how to make yourself up?
When first writing this book in 2017 I didn't really have that as a set goal, but today, in 2020, I am an examined makeup artist. I took a ten week course and learned so much about how to do makeup on a face different than mine.

Do you prefer colorful makeup (lipstick, eye shadow) or a more natural look?
It really depends on my mood when applying my makeup. I love both color explosions and feature enhancing neutral looks.

If you had only ONE product to use before you left home, what would it be?
I think I would choose an eyebrow pencil, concealer or mascara. Wow, that's a hard one.

Questions to help you:

What are your best tricks for foundation to stay put during the day?
Know your skin and skin type and as with your skin care, tailor your makeup after that. What do you want your foundation to do? Hydrate? Mattify? Be long-wearing? There is no foundation that suits everyone. Try different techniques––baking, applying powder under your foundation, patting your setting spray in with a damp makeup sponge. Finding your perfect recipe takes time and will only be better if you try different options.

How to find the right foundation shade?
I think it is easiest to go to the makeup store without makeup and test the colors lightly on your chin/jaw. Your hand/arm is most likely not the same shade as your face. Whatever blends in seamlessly on your jaw/chin/neck will be the right shade for you. A plus is if you know your undertone so you can narrow down your options to only warm, cool or neutral tones.

Do you have any tricks to make an everyday makeup look a little extra and festive?
The best trick I have is either shimmer or glitter. Shimmer on the eyelid or a little glitter in the inner corner of the eye gives any kind of everyday makeup a festive look. If you want to keep your eyes to the bare minimum, pair them with a bold lip or some

Makeup

false eyelashes. That also instantly amps up the festive feel of your makeup.

Tips on getting a good eyeliner?
Breathe, practice, find inner calm, practice, say a prayer, and hope for the best. Also, get to know your eye shape. Following a tutorial for large eyes with a ton of lid space won't help you if you have hooded eyes.

Tips on getting a good eyeliner?
Breathe, practice, find inner calm, practice, say a prayer, and hope for the best.

I just tried baking and then took a selfie with flash. It was completely white around the eyes of the picture, and I don't understand why.
You have probably used a so-called HD powder that reflects harsh light and makes the powder fully visible in the photo. Avoid HD powders if you know that photos will be taken with flash. HD powder is best suited for daylight and on video.

How do you pluck your eyebrows properly?
Always pluck under the brow and do not care much about the hairs that grow above, if they are not coarse. By plucking underneath, you keep a nice arch and avoid the temptation of plucking until you leave the bathroom with the brows everyone and their mothers had in the 90's.

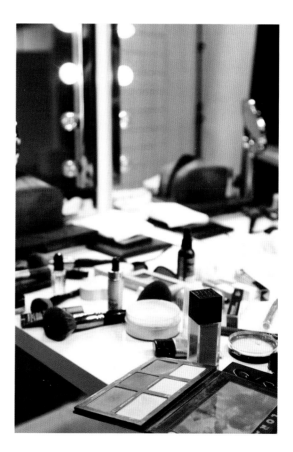

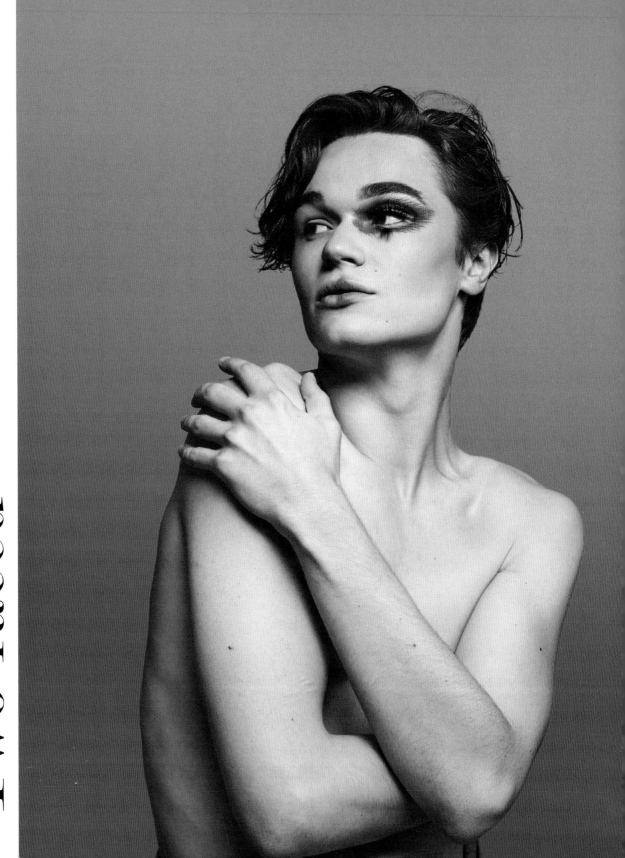

Two faced

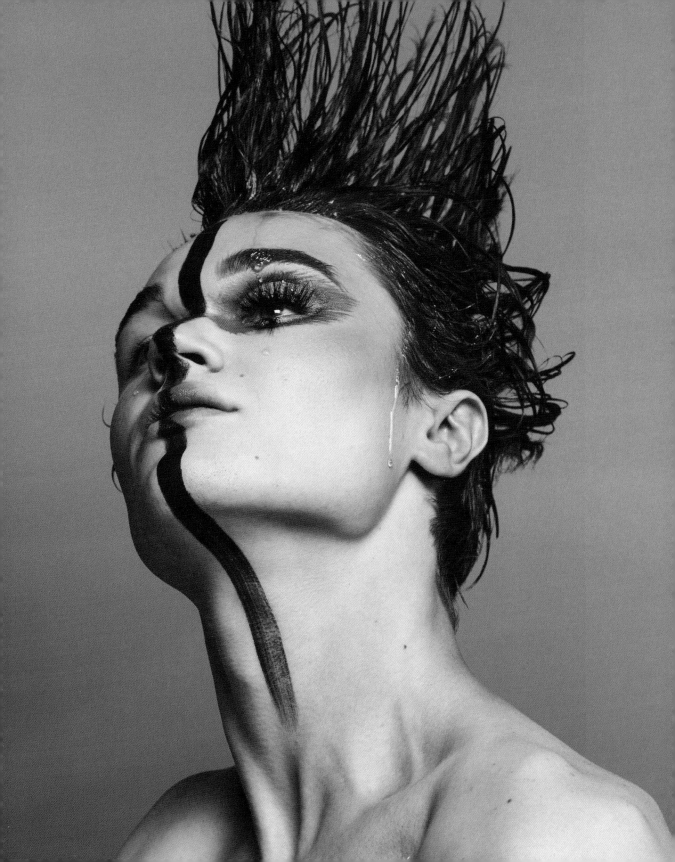

Glossary

baking: A technique used both to brighten up and fix concealer, which is to apply a thick layer of powder on top of the concealer and allow it to be absorbed. Excess powder is then brushed off.

bronzer: Immediately gives your face a fresh, sun-kissed look. Apply with a large, soft, and fluffy brush on the face, wherever you get sun first. Often used to compliment your shading and to warm up your complexion.

brow pomade: A creamy waterproof wax, often used with a narrow brush to fill in brows.

concealer: Available many forms such as liquid, cream, and powder and is used primarily to cover blemishes and dark circles in your face. If used in a lighter shade it also highlights and shapes your face.

consistencies: Liquid, mousse, powder, stick, cream, whipped, to name a few.

contouring: Also called shading. A technique to shape the face with cool shades. You apply this to areas you want to shape or deepen.

cut crease: An eyeshadow technique where a sharp line is applied above the natural crease to give the illusion of a bigger eyelid.

eyeliner: A line that is mainly applied right above the upper lash line to extend and enhance the eyes.

false lashes: Artificial eyelashes attached to the roots of the natural lashes. Available in both strips and single lashes. Reusable.

foundation: Base for your makeup that provides coverage and evens out your skin tone.

highlighter: Used, for example, on the cheekbones, under the eye, under the eyebrow, and along the nostril to create glow. Available both in powder, as a cream, shimmering or matte.

kohl pencil: Soft eye pencil used to contour, line and/or smoke out the eyes. Provides softer lines compared to liquid eyeliner and can be blended.

lip gloss: Available both transparent and with pigment. Use either alone or with lipstick for extra gloss.

lip pencil: Used to outline and enhance the lip shape, as a base before lipstick or gloss.

mixing liquid: A transparent, liquid product used to mix products (for example, securing glitter or loose pigment), to make a product waterproof or to make a dry product more creamy.

pack on: Put on a lot of a powder product, such as eye shadow or baking powder.

primer: Evens out, hydrates, blurs, mattifies (depending on the properties of the product) the skin and keeps the makeup in place for a long time. Apply primer after day cream but before foundation.

setting spray: By using a setting spray on your face as the last step in your makeup, the base, the natural oils in the skin, and the powder are fixed. Powder products look more like skin and makeup lasts longer.

spoolie brush: A small, twisted brush head that separates and shapes eyebrows. Similar to a mascara brush.

waterline: The eyelid edge closest to the whites and covered by tear fluid.

July 2018

<u>Thanks!</u>

As I write this, the book has not been released yet, but I know that not all the reactions will be positive. My made up face can sometimes be incredibly provocative. And that is understandable; I mean, who wouldn't be provoked by a contour as seamlessly blended as mine?

Jokes aside, thank you to everyone who fights daily for their and others' rights in society. You are heroes forging paths in a forest that's hard for many people to find their way out of.

With this book, I want to pay tribute to makeup, teach my knowledge that I gathered up along the way during my few years as a makeup enthusiast, tell my stories, and hopefully be able to change the views about people who use makeup and don't fit in with society's image of who should wear makeup.

Mom, Dad, and my sister: I love you and am so grateful for your support, both around the book and in my life. You let go of the handlebars on my bike when I learned to ride, but kept walking beside it. The same way you do in my life. Thanks.

To my friends, thank you for being yourselves and adding what you do to my life, and for all the piercing shrieks you erupted with when I nervously showed images from the day's photoshoot; my ego is satisfied for the rest of my life. You are the best friends a person could have for so many reasons, not just for your appreciative shrieks.

I have always wanted to inspire the world even as I change it, and, Mom, I think I have found the meaning of life.

December 2020

Two and a half years has passed since I wrote the words on the left, and updating this book has been such an emotional journey. I have changed so much as a person, I have come to terms with my true authentic self and I am now just beginning to become who I truly am. Writing this my eyes fill up with tears—I am just so ready to leave this feeling of being trapped and stuck behind me. I know that the world can be a dark place, and yes, I am scared, but the positive aspect of coming out as the woman that I am is way too big for my fears to hold me back.

I yet again want to thank everyone who is fighting for their and others' rights in society. You are so important and pave the way for so many, such as myself, and I hope to be able to do the same.

What I wrote in 2018 still stands—to my family, thank you, I love you and can thank you enough for your support. Same goes to my friends, I don't know where I'd be without you.

After a period of massive confusion and loss of hope, I feel that I am finally building myself up again to change the world, little by little, and this time, as my true authentic self.

I hope this book marks the beginning to those of you who always wanted to improve your makeup skills, brings joy, knowledge, understanding, hope and is a fine addition to your makeup station, coffee table or shelf.

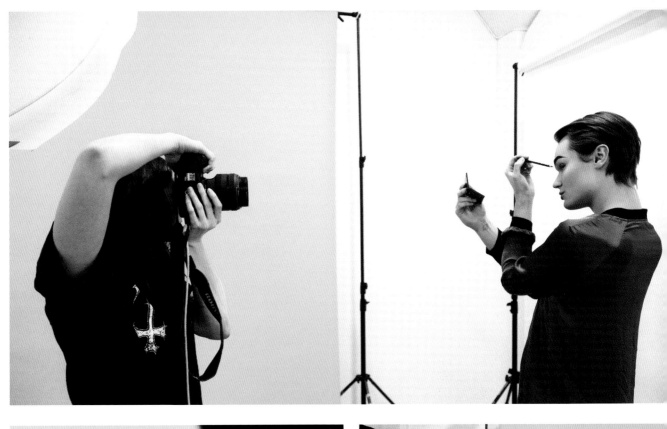
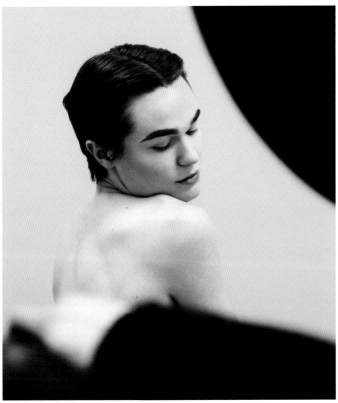
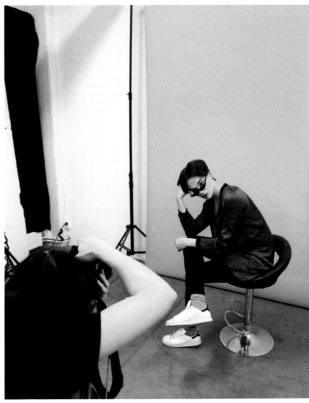